First published January 2019
Text © Yin Pilates, 2019
Published by LettsStretch Publications
www.anthonylett.com
Modelling & Photography: Kenyi Diaz
Graphic Design: Angela Shi & Kenyi Diaz
Cover Image: Pawel Kuczynski

National Library of Australia Cataloguing-in-Publication entry

Creator:	Lett, Anthony, author.
Title:	Disrupting Text Neck: Your guide to managing neck pain, headache, stress and insomnia / Anthony Lett
ISBN:	9781795619837 (paperback)
Subjects:	Pilates method.
	Health.
	Physical fitness.
Dewey Number:	613.7192

All rights reserved. No part of this book may be reproduced or transmitted in any form or by any means, electronic or mechanical, including photocopying, recording or by any information storage and retrieval system, without written permission from the publisher, except for the inclusion of brief quotations in a review.

The author and publisher have taken care in the preparation of this book but make no expressed or implied warranty of any kind and assume no responsibility for errors or omissions. No liability is assumed for incidental or consequential damages in connection with or arising out of the use of the information or programs contained herein.

Disrupting Text Neck

Your guide to managing neck pain, headache, stress and insomnia

Anthony Lett

Anthony

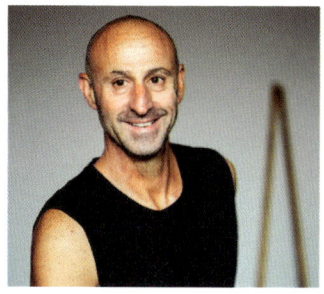

… is a StretchFit studio owner, teacher, educator and writer originally from Melbourne Australia. Anthony teaches workshops globally on the material from his books titled *Innovations in Pilates* and *StretchFit*. Anthony was the Director of Advanced Education for BASI Pilates and has qualifications in philosophy, sports science, exercise medicine and clinical anatomy. Anthony has presented his workshops and keynote addresses in over 25 countries and is a leading creative thinker in the Pilates industry. Anthony's six books contain fascinating world-first 3D Pilates graphics and merge practices from osteopathy, physiotherapy and Yoga with traditional Pilates repertoire. Anthony also created the first *Pilates Anatomy* certification course, as well as the first 3D printed Pilates reformer. *Pilates Anatomy* involves three-dimensional anatomy video, creation of muscles on skeletons, and exploration of functional anatomy in the Pilates studio. Anthony and his wife, Kenyi, operate a StretchFit studio in Fitzroy Melbourne and teach retreats in Bali Indonesia.

http://anthonylett.com

Kenyi

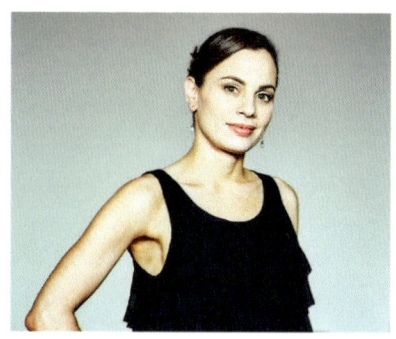

… is a professional Pilates instructor originally from Venezuela, with a background in dance, and training in classical and contemporary Pilates. Kenyi began teaching Pilates in 2004. Kenyi has taught Innovations in Pilates workshops in Australia, Asia, Europe, the UK, South Africa and South America. A skilled graphic artist, Kenyi designed and co-authored all of the *Innovations in Pilates* materials including books, ebooks and video production. Kenyi is pursuing an academic interest in human nutrition; in particular, eating for health and wellbeing, for sports performance, and in the growing area of "food as medicine". In 2018, Kenyi released a book on the Pilates Wunda chair.

diazkenyi@gmail.com
www.kenyidiaz.com

Contents

Part A 7

    Introduction 8

    For geeks 12

    How often to stretch 16

    In summary 17

Part B: The Stretches 19

    Introduction 20

    Lateral flexion 21

    Flexion A: Chin to chest 24

    Flexion B: Atlanto-occipital 'nodding' flexion 24

    Extension 26

    Rotation 29

    Vertebrobasilar insufficiency 34

Additional Variations 37

    The combination variation 38

    Flexion of the entire spine 40

    Seated rotation of the entire spine 44

    Thoracic extension 47

Quick Reference Guide 49

    Neck flexion 50

    The combination variation 51

Neck lateral flexion 52

Neck rotation 53

Neck extension and rotation 54

Jaw extension 55

Conclusion 56

Part A

Introduction

The purpose of this book is mostly practical. Most of the content involves teaching you how to release accumulated tension in the muscles of the head and neck safely and simply.

Before we get to the practical work though, let's have a brief look at the background to "text neck," including its recent emergence, the changes that it brings about in your body and some of the underlying anatomical and biomechanical factors that create it. For those of you who are not anatomically minded, I have put the more complex anatomical and biomechanical information under a subheading titled "For geeks." You may skip this information in the interests of saving your neck from further tension!

The Stretches are presented in two parts. The first is more detailed. The "Quick Reference Guide" that follows consists of dot points to remind you what to do, perhaps in the middle of doing it. My suggestion is that you read about and practice the stretches in greater detail first and then use the quick reference guide when you feel more familiar with each stretch.

What is Text Neck?

Text Neck is classed as an overuse syndrome or a repetitive stress injury to the neck caused by holding your head in a forward and downward position for extended periods of time. When holding your head in this position, excessive amounts of tension are created in the deep muscles of your neck and across the shoulders causing both acute and chronic neck pain, shoulder pain, upper back pain, headache, jaw pain, insomnia and increased thoracic curvature or "kyphosis."

Text neck is a very recent phenomenon and is due to the increasing hours spent on handheld devices such as personal computers, smartphones, e-readers and tablets.

Mismatch Diseases

Many of the illnesses and conditions that we confront today are what evolutionary biologists call "mismatch diseases": ...Conditions or maladies that occur because our bodies (or necks) are poorly or inadequately adapted to the environments in which we now live. So, mismatch diseases are conditions that are more modern in the sense that they're more prevalent, or even novel or more severe, because we don't live in the way in which our bodies are adapted. Text neck is one such condition, along with for example, eating vast quantities of sugar and moving an average of just 500 meters per day. We simply have not evolved to sit and "turtle neck" for hours on end day after day. The result is a new and novel condition now reaching epidemic proportions.

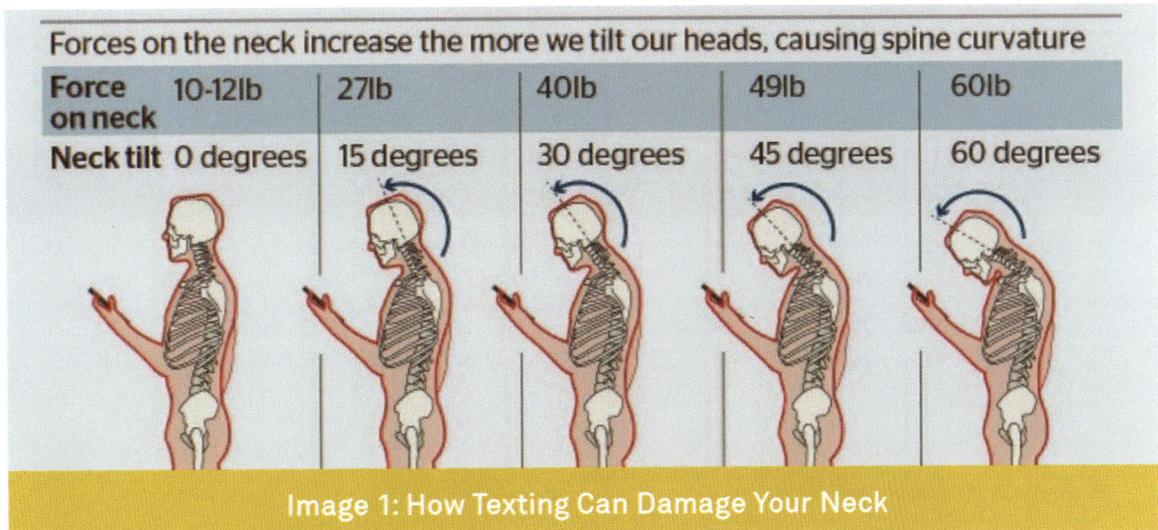

Image 1: How Texting Can Damage Your Neck

What Exactly Causes Text Neck?

When in an upright posture the ears are aligned with the center of your shoulders and the weight of the average head exerts approximately 10-12lbs of force through the muscles of the neck. But when your head is moved forward by one 1 inch away from this neutral position, the weight of your head dramatically increases as the image above demonstrates. Approximately 6 times as much force can be generated! That is the same weight as an average 8 year old, or six Ten-pin bowling balls!!! (See image one)

Consequences

Of course, your neck was not designed to load the equivalent of an eight-year-old child across it while staring at a screen for hours on a daily basis. The outcome of such physical stress goes something like this: (Please excuse the slightly exclusory medical language. In any case, you'll get the picture.)

- Stress (physical or psychological) causes biochemical changes in the brain, increasing neural excitability
- Postural changes follow in muscles, involving increased tone, retarding circulation, increasing calcium, lactic and hyaluronic acid accumulation
- Local contractile activity in muscles is increased which shortens and tenses muscle bundles
- Sustained metabolic activity in muscles leads to vasoconstriction, lack of oxygen, reduction in removal of metabolic waste, toxic build up, pain, tenderness. This becomes a self perpetuating loop-pain creates more hypertonicity & pain.

- Local pressure builds up involving waste products &chemicals causing spasm, local and referred pain.
- After days or weeks, fibrotic changes in connective tissue will follow.
- Tendons and insertions of hypertonic muscles become stressed. Tendon pain and periosteal pain result.
- Muscle imbalances begin to emerge- chain reactions of dysfunction. A process develops in which some muscles will be used inappropriately as they compensate for weaker or restricted muscles, leading to adaptive movements.
- Osteo- Arthritic changes can occur in advanced cases in the joints involved.

Psychological Stress

It should also be noted that a consequence of our immersion into a world of 24/7 connectivity is significant psychological stress too, with many of the same physical manifestations as in the list above. The expectation that we will be available 24/7 has spawned a new acronym called "FOMO" or the Fear of Missing Out, and it is well known to all of us. Missing a social event, a job promotion or an important meeting or conference call that often occurs outside of conventional working hours can create significant anxiety and muscle tension.

What ever it is, psychological stress results in an increase in sympathetic arousal, (the sympathetic nervous system is a branch of the autonomic nervous system) known commonly as the "fight or flight" response. **This elevates muscle tension throughout the body.** If a region like the neck, already suffering increased activation from the physical stress of "text neck," experiences even greater arousal due to psychological factors, it will be the first place to signal increased tension and pain. Hence, the physical aspects of text neck and the often-associated psychological factors combine to produce a neck that can seriously affect our wellbeing.

In addition, the 'startle response' doesn't help matters. Stress physiology studies demonstrate that the universal response to acute stress includes activation of the extensor muscles of the neck -the ones that pull it backwards and poke out the chin. Known as the 'startle response', this is thought to be a remnant of our quadruped past, when we would hunch our shoulders to protect the vital organs of the neck and tilt our head back in order to see our enemy.

In the field of mind-body medicine, it is a very well-established fact that repeatedly becoming stressed eventually becomes damaging. "Stress" writes Sapolsky in his modern classic *Why Zebras Don't Get Ulcers* "increases your risk of getting diseases that make you sick, or if you have a disease, stress increases the risk of your defences being overwhelmed by the disease." Modern stress related diseases include heart disease, some types of cancer, cerebrovascular disorders, high cholesterol and type two diabetes. When continually activated the fight or flight response increases our vulnerability to depression, the speed at which we age and how well our memories work. One of the first books on the subject of stress and mind/ body medicine was called *The Relaxation Response* by doctor Herb Benson. It can be found online and it's a gem. Readers interested in stress physiology and its management are well advised to start with this one, and Sapolsky's book above.

Treatment and Self Management

Text neck is generally conservatively managed by some kind of physical therapy. The main aims of treatment are to reduce the tension within neck muscles, reduce pain within the neck and shoulder region and address the postures that aggravate symptoms. The work in this text provides a similar approach except that you will be learning to perform it yourself. A self-management approach provides a sense of self efficacy and being in control permits a degree of relaxation that is rarely experienced during treatment in the hands of someone else. Relaxation, as the information above spells out, is an absolutely central aspect of effective treatment. Self-management also equips you with the tools to practice anytime without the often-considerable costs of treatment.

The positive news is that if we do not stress ourselves beyond a certain threshold, our capacity for positive adaptation is quite miraculous. In fact we can reverse many of the stress responses outlined above by practicing the simple exercises following shortly. Reducing muscle tension and inducing the 'relaxation response' – the opposite of the chronic fight or flight response so prevalent today – can be as simple as maintaining a weekly practice of stretching and relaxion. In addition, if you can avail your self of the services of a good ergonomist to evaluate your daily work environment, you will reduce the overall stress load that you are exposed to. The resulting freedom from pain and discomfort will make a serious difference to your life. Do the work consistently and the changes will come. If your pain is not totally reduced, at least your ability to manage and control its severity will be increased. For anyone who suffers chronic pain the suggestion that you can have some control over it is welcome news.

A note on anatomy, kinesiology and biomechanics

To "treat" oneself effectively it is unnecessary to name every muscle being affected. In fact, the effort to do so might create an acute text neck response! For example, in the first lateral flexion stretch below the following muscles are stretched: upper trapezius muscle, rotatores, intertransversarii, interspinalis, multifidus, rectus capitis posterior major and minor, obliquus capitis inferior and superior, semispinalis capitis, longissimus capitis, scalenus medius, rectus capitis lateralis, splenius capitis, and sternocleidomastoid.

Rather than naming all these muscles, what's important is that by exploring all the stretches you locate your tight regions and continue to stretch them until your range of movement increases and your pain is reduced. This is what matters. Consequently, the next section "For geeks" really is just that- a section that might only be of interest to those who practice bodywork of some kind, who teach, or who enjoy mechanical analysis. If it's not for you, skip over it and move on to the final part of the introduction on how often to stretch, and how to practice "contract/relax" stretching.

For Geeks

The anatomy, kinesiology and biomechanics of text neck

Nearly 30 pairs of muscles cross the craniocervical region. This mass of muscle also serves to protect the cervical viscera and blood vessels, intervertebral discs, apophyseal joints, and neural tissues. The muscles can be classified into three rough categories.

The first includes the muscles that act exclusively within the craniocervical region called the suboccipital muscles. See **Image two**. These muscles are dedicated to providing precise control over the two highly specialized joints at the top of the spine which are given unique names. At C1 is the "atlas" and C2 the "axis." See Image three. A fine level of control is essential for optimal positioning of the eyes, ears, and nose. Many of the suboccipital muscle contractions are primarily reflexive in nature and linked to neural centers that help coordinate vision and associated righting and postural reactions of the head and neck.

A second group could be likened to the 'core" muscles of the lumbar region for example, which do not produce large scale movements of the spine but instead control the fine movements of one vertebra in relation to its neighbor. Much of the muscular stabilization of the craniocervical region is accomplished by these relatively short, segmented muscles such as the multifidi, rotatores, longus colli, capitis, and interspinalis muscles. With relatively short fibers and multiple bony attachments, these muscles exert a fine, coordinated control of the stability in the region.

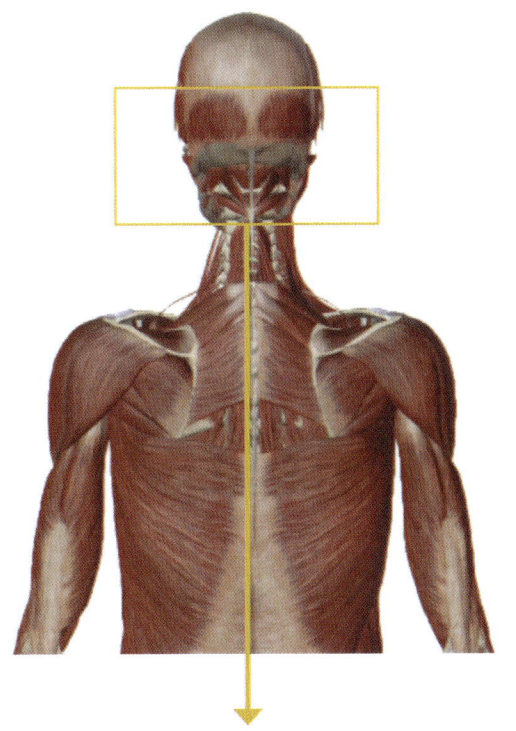

Image 2

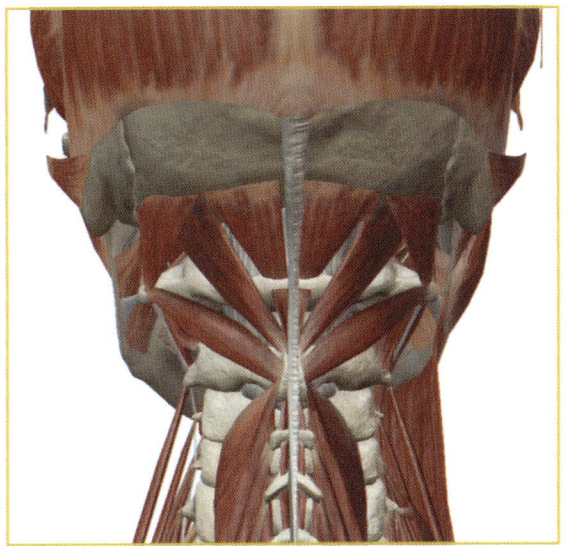

This stability is augmented by a third group of longer and typically thicker muscles, including the scalenes, sternocleidomastoid, levator scapula, semispinalis capitis and cervicis, and trapezius. When needed, these muscles form an extensive and strong guy-wire system that ensures vertical stability, most notably in frontal and sagittal planes, as well as producing extensive and well-coordinated movements of the head and neck. As in the thoracic and lumbar regions, the co-contraction of flexor and extensor muscles counterbalances, and as a consequence vertically stabilizes the region.

This third group of muscles are anchored inferiorly to several different structures: the sternum, clavicle, ribs, scapula, and vertebral column. Consequently, these bony structures themselves must be stabilized by other muscles, such as the lower trapezius and subclavius, to secure the scapula and clavicle, respectively.

In fact, movement of the craniocervical region requires muscular interactions that extend well into the trunk and lower extremities. For example, the activation of the right and left oblique abdominal muscles provides much of the force/torque needed to stabilize the thoracic region, required as a structural foundation for the craniocervical region.

Image 3

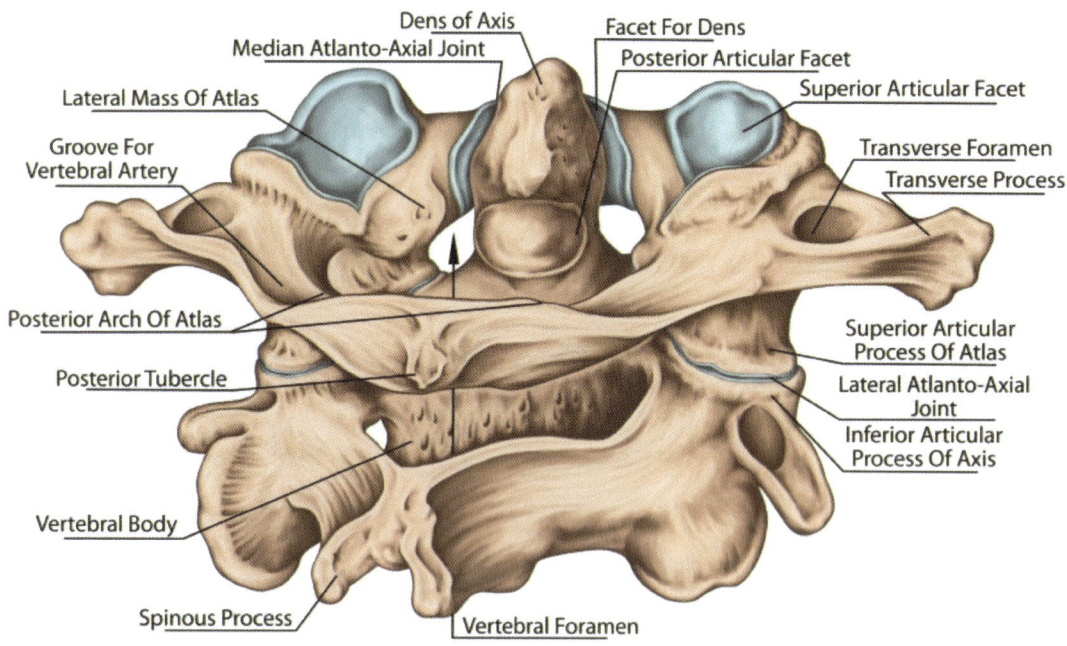

Image 4

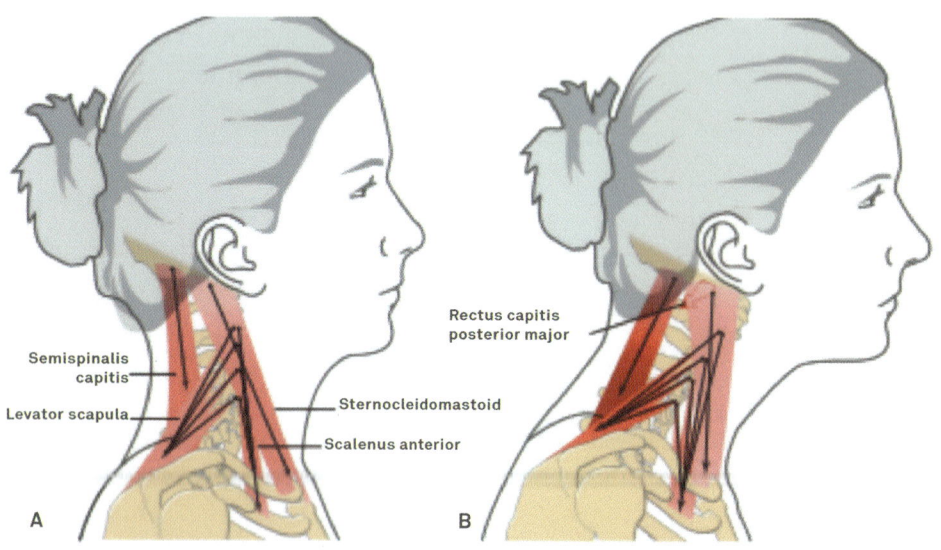

Muscular Imbalance Associated with Chronic Forward Head Posture

The ideal posture shown in Image 4-A depicts an optimally balanced craniocervical "guy-wire" system. Excessive muscular tension in any of the muscles, however, can disrupt the vertical stability of the region. Text Neck is one such disruption with a chronic forward head posture, involving excessive protraction of the craniocervical region.

Habitual forward head posture can occur for at least two different reasons. First, severe hyperextension of the neck can injure anterior muscles, such as the sternocleidomastoid, longus colli, and scalenus anterior. As a result, chronic spasm in the excessively strained muscles translates the head forward, resulting in excessive flexion, especially at the cervicothoracic junction.

A clinical sign often associated with forward head posturing is a realignment of the sternocleidomastoid within the sagittal plane. The cranial end of the muscle, normally aligned posterior to the sternoclavicular joint, shifts anteriorly with the head to a position directly above the sternoclavicular joint (compare A with B).

A second cause of a chronic forward head posture may be related to a progressive shortening of several anterior neck muscles. One such scenario involves purposely protracting the craniocervical region to improve visual contact with objects manipulated in front of the body. This activity is typical when viewing a computer screen or a television. This position, if adopted for an extended period, may alter the functional resting length of the muscles, eventually transforming the forward posture into a person's "natural" posture.

Regardless of the factors that predispose a person to a chronic forward head posture, the posture itself stresses extensor muscles, such as the levator scapula and semispinalis capitis (see Figure 4-B). A suboccipital muscle, such as the rectus capitis posterior major, may become fatigued as a result of its prolonged extension activity required to "level" the head and eyes. Over time, increased muscular stress throughout the entire craniocervical region can lead to localized and painful muscle spasms, or "trigger points," common in the levator scapula and suboccipital muscles. This condition is often associated with headaches and radiating pain into the scalp and temporomandibular joints.

How often to stretch

Neck stretching is often employed as a curative practice, but in my experience it is best used as a preventative measure.

The stretches here ought to be practised in the *absence* of headaches or pain, or with great gentleness at its onset, but not in the midst of a debilitating episode. Practising the stretches during a headache or pain episode will often exacerbate the symptoms. It is better to wait until the headache or pain has subsided and then practise this sequence of stretches up to every day or two. Once this becomes routine, you will find yourself a master at managing your own pain and stress responses.

Contract/Relax

CR is called a neuromuscular technique because it uses the nervous system and isometric muscle contraction (isometric meaning 'without movement') to trick muscles into releasing tension.

The three step process is simple. First, move your head to a position where you feel a moderate stretch. Let's call this the point of tension, or POT. Hold the position for five deep breaths. Second, isometrically 'activate' (contract) the muscles that are being stretched. Do this by pressing your head back against a barrier with no more than 30% of your maximum force for five seconds. The barrier in this series will be your free hand. Relax and take a breath in. Third, on the breath out, restretch and move to a new POT, holding this final position for ten deep breaths.

In Summary:

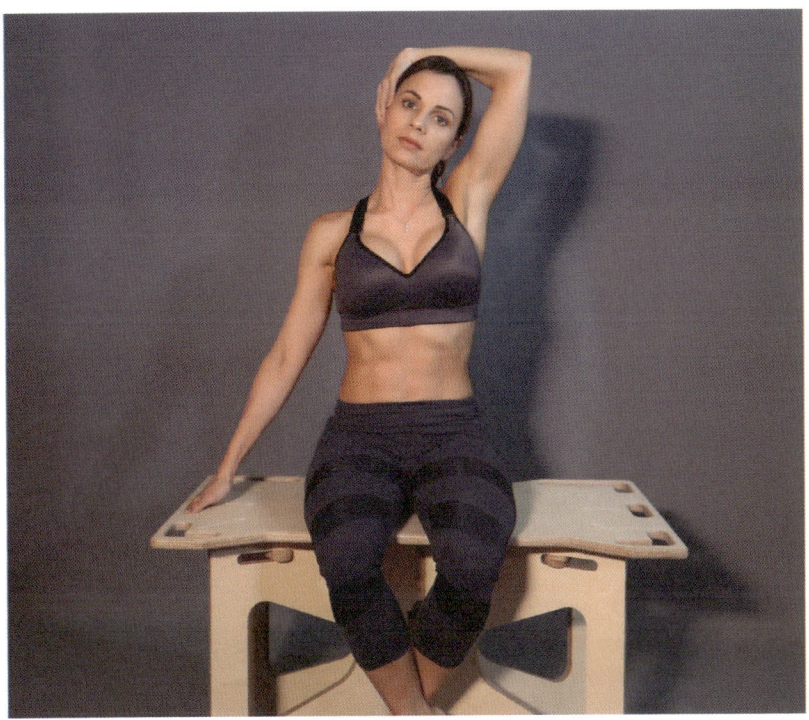

1 Move to the initial POT for five breaths. Approximately 5 out of ten in intensity.

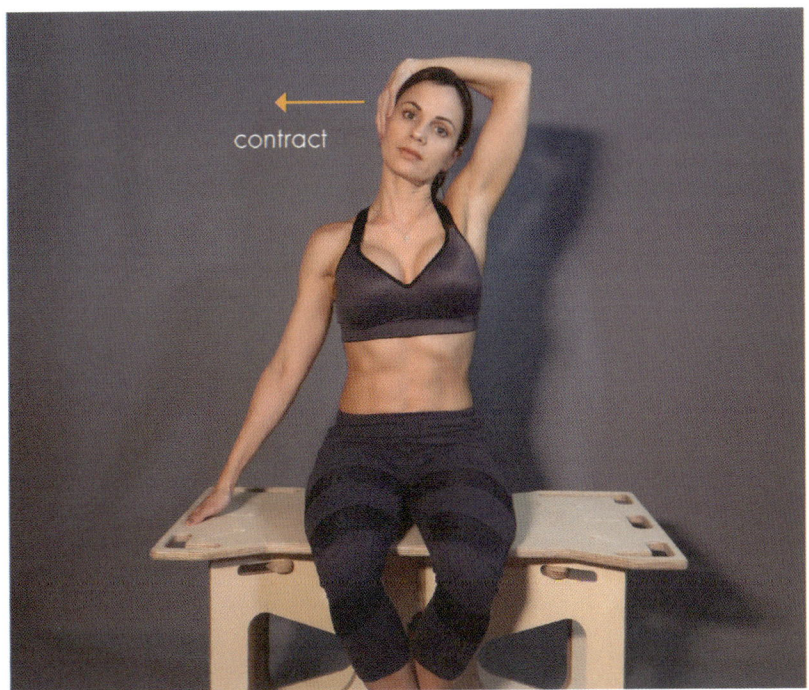

2 Contract for 5 seconds, using 30% of maximal force at most without any movement occuring.

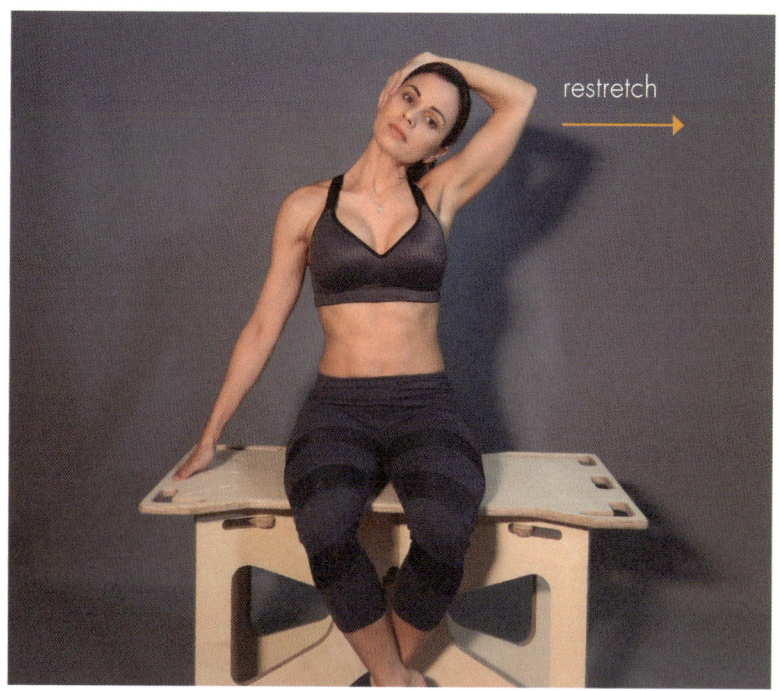

3. Relax and stretch further to the new POT for ten breaths. Don't expect huge re-stretch movement. One centimeter is considerable.

References

Boyd-Clark LC, Briggs CA, Galea MP: Muscle spindle distribution, morphology, and density in longus colli and multifidus muscles of the cervical spine, Spine 27:694-701, 2002.

Chaffin DB, Andersson GBJ: Occupational Biomechanics, 2nd ed, New York, 1991, John Wiley and Sons.

Deng YC, Goldsmith W: Response of a human head/neck/upper-torso replica to dynamic loading—I. Physical model, J Biomech 20:471-486, 1987.

Fujishiro K, Weaver JL, Heaney CA, et al: The effect of ergonomic interventions in healthcare facilities on musculoskeletal disorders, Am J Ind Med 48:338-347, 2005.

Part B:
The Stretches

Introduction

The basic movements of the neck are **flexion, extension, lateral flexion** and **rotation**.

These four movements, and some of them in combination, make up this text. Placing your fingers in the slots of the "Neck Deck" and leaning in the direction of the arrows will ensure that all of these movements are practiced. If you don't have a "Neck Deck" a chair will suffice. Place your fingers under the edge and follow the instructions.

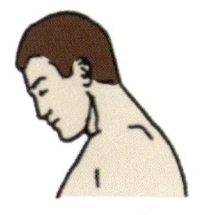 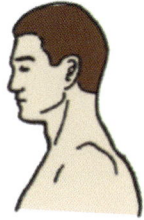 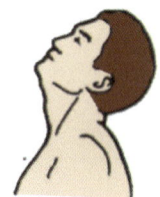 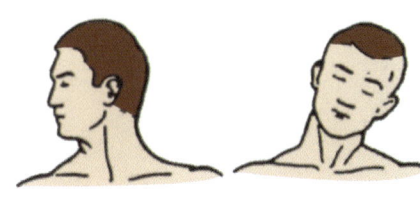

Flexion   Neutral   Extension   Rotation   Lateral flexion

Lateral Flexion

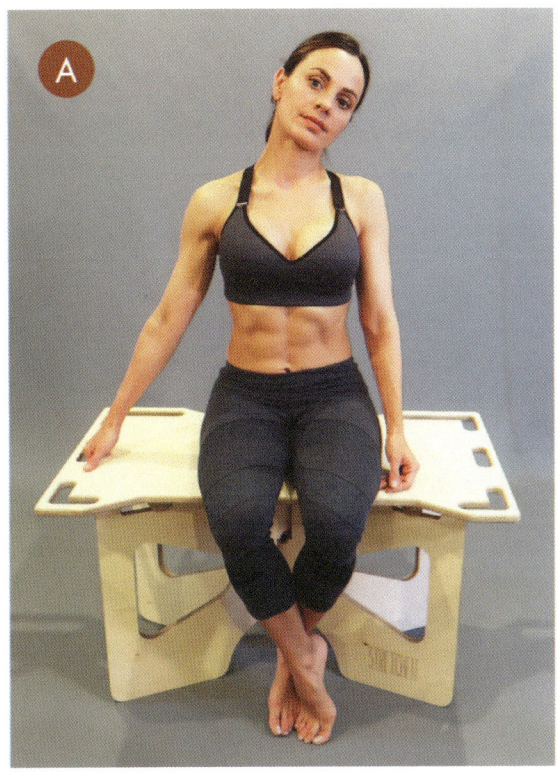

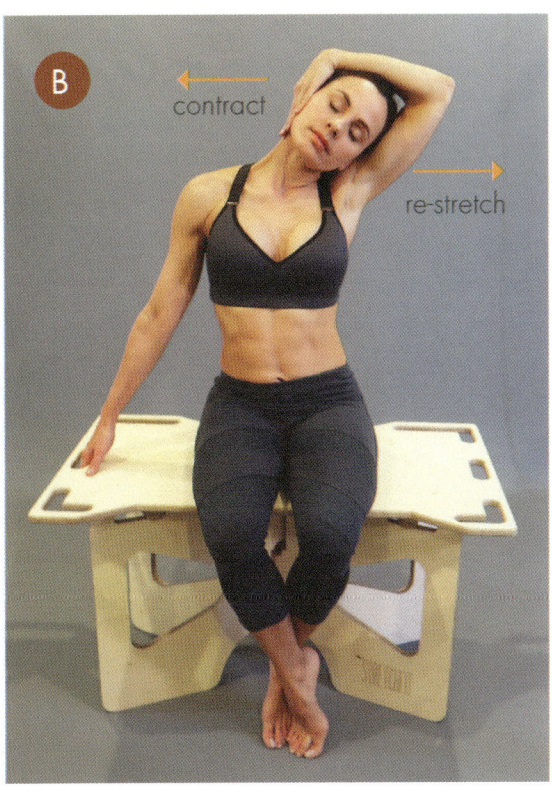

Background

Let's begin with lateral flexion, or side-bending of the neck. Tightness in side-bending ability is common and may contribute to abnormal scapulohumeral rhythm, shoulder impingement syndrome, tension headache and various other complaints.

'Normal' range of movement here is between 40 and 45 degrees from the neutral position. The neutral position is where your head is positioned precisely between your shoulders without any deviation.

How to stretch (Image A)

Sit up tall and feel the weight of both sit bones (ischial tuberosities) on the seat. Sit so that you can reach through the slot with your arm, keeping both sit bones on the deck.

Lean away from the restraining hand, ensuring that when you do so the shoulder is drawn down away from your ear. If you are sitting too close to the restraining hand, the side of your bottom will lift. If this occurs, adjust your sitting position.

Lean away and reach your free hand up and over your head. Spread your fingers onto your neck and rest the weight of your head on your arm (Image B). Relax!

Make a body scan: draw your awareness from your restraining hand, up your arm, through the biceps to the shoulder. How much tension can you let go of? Can you relax the grip a little, and let your shoulders drop? I bet you can. Hold this position for five breaths and try not to move.

Text Neck 21

Lateral Flexion

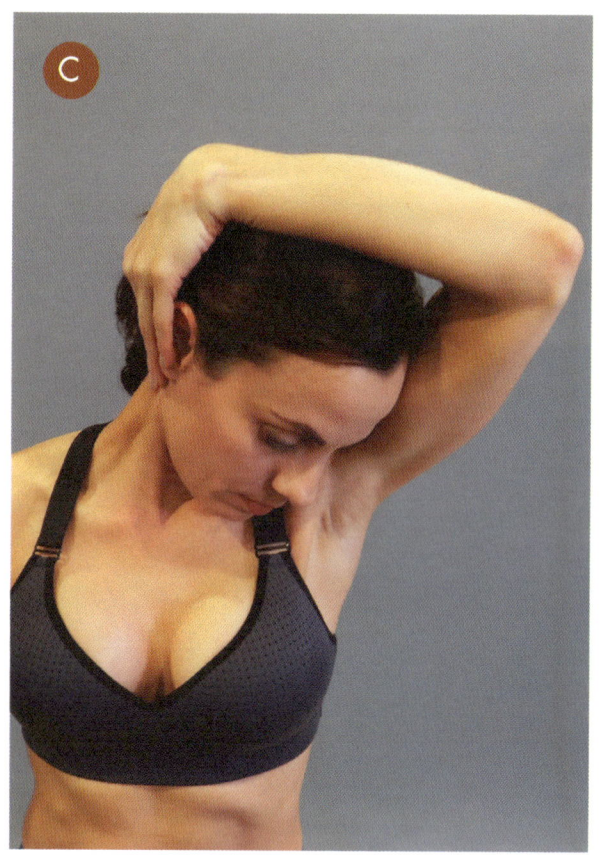

How to contract (Image B)

Press your head back into the hand on your head towards your starting position (see arrow). Use up to 30% of your maximum effort but start with as little as 5%. Notice the difference in feeling between the relaxed neck and the neck as it develops tension. This awareness is an important element in self-management. Press your head into your hand for five seconds without allowing any movement to occur, and then relax.

Restretch (Image B)

Relax again and take a deep breath in. On the breath out do two things: lean further from the restraining hand, and pull a little on your head with your fingers. Tensioning the skin with your fingers will increase the stretch sensation. Be sure to lean directly sideways for the moment. Hold the stretch for ten deep breaths and let your body go limp. Closing your eyes might assist with relaxation, 'Soften your eyes in their sockets,' as my yoga teacher used to say. To complete the stretch, roll your chin down to your chest and then return your head slowly back to the neutral position.

Variations (Image C)

While in the above stretch, rotate your head toward your right armpit. This will move the stretch sensation from the side of the neck toward the back of the neck, on the side that you are leaning away from. This combines **lateral flexion** with **rotation**.

Major Muscles Stretched

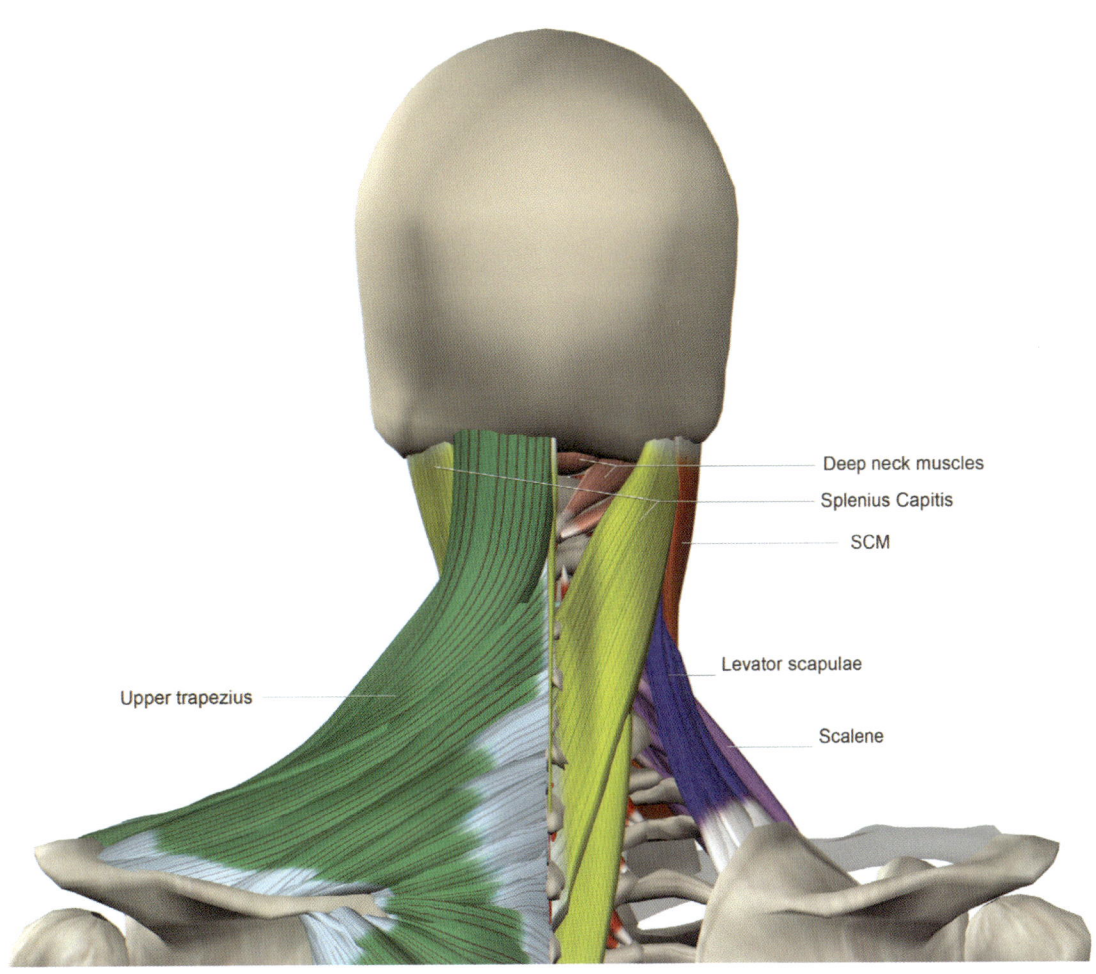

Flexion A: Chin to Chest

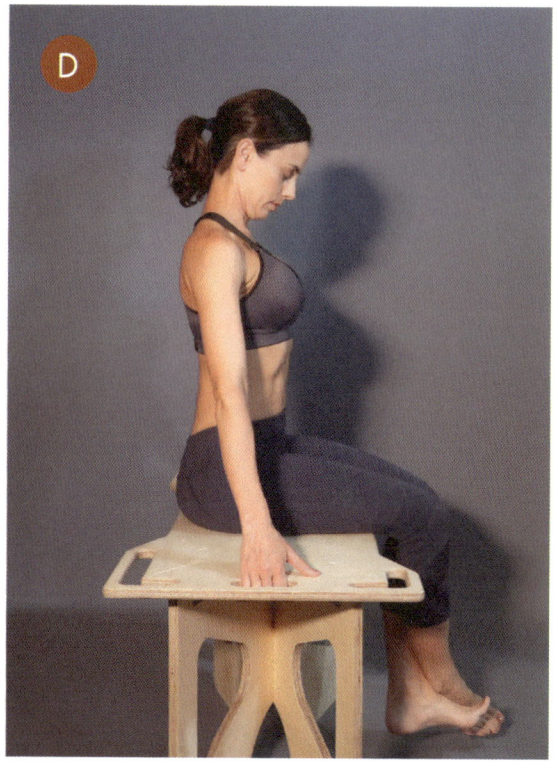

Background

This stretch involves **flexion** of the neck. There are two ways of flexing the neck. One involves taking the chin toward the chest (see Image E), which stretches the large bulk of muscles running posteriorly along all of the cervical vertebrae, and the second involves tucking the chin back toward the neck (See Image D). This is known as atlanto-occipital flexion and occurs mostly at the level of C1 and C2. Try both movements, because it is possible that you are tight in both regions, or one and not the other.

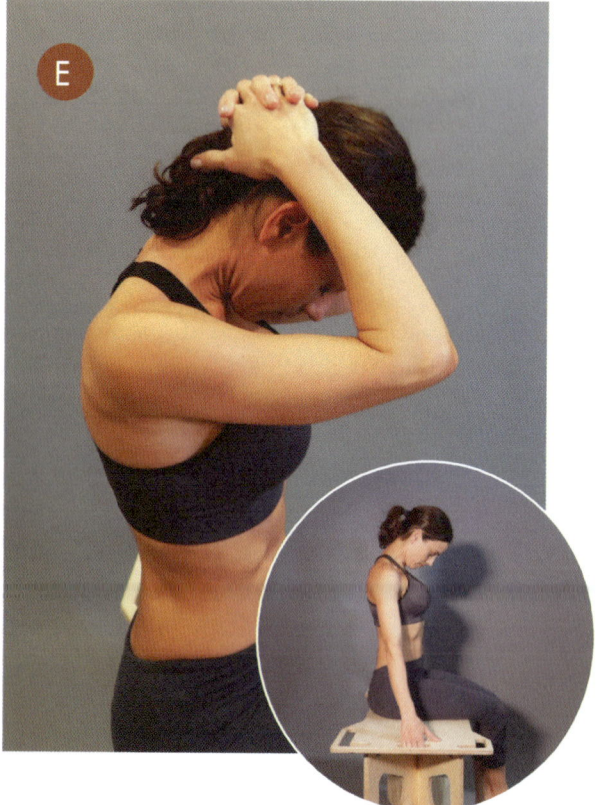

How to stretch (Image E)

Sit up tall, with your weight distributed evenly onto both sit bones. Take your chin toward your chest and then place your hands gently onto the back of your head as pictured (Image E). Take as much of the weight of your hands and arms onto your head as necessary to give you a stretch.

As usual, take a deep breath in and relax. Try not to bend the whole of your spine, just the region above your shoulders. Do not force the issue. Stretching is about cajoling, not coercing. Pull gently on your scalp as if you are going to drag the hair from the back of your head onto the top of your head. Tensioning the scalp will increase the stretch.

Flexion A: Chin to Chest

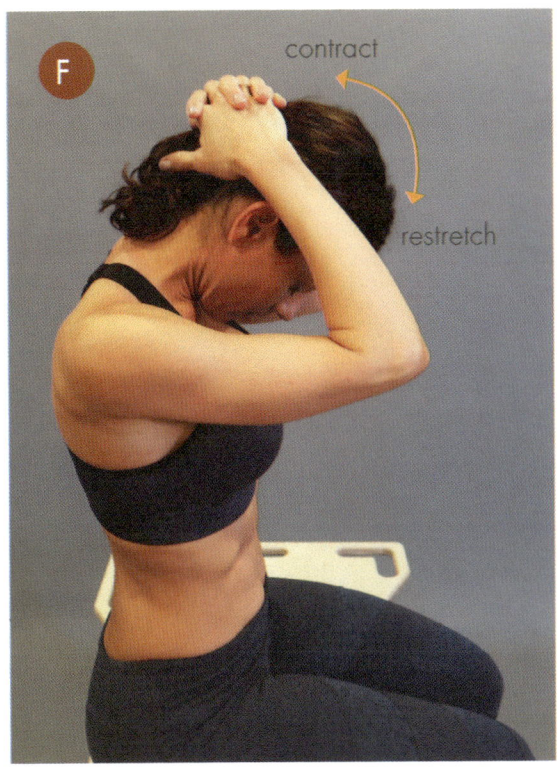

How to contract (Image F)

Press the whole of your head back into your hands for five seconds. As always, start with minimal force and increase to about 30% of your maximum.

Restretch (Image F)

Take a deep breath in. On the breath out take your chin toward your chest. Use your arms to apply a little more force, and again pull on your scalp. Relax your shoulders and hold for up to ten breaths.

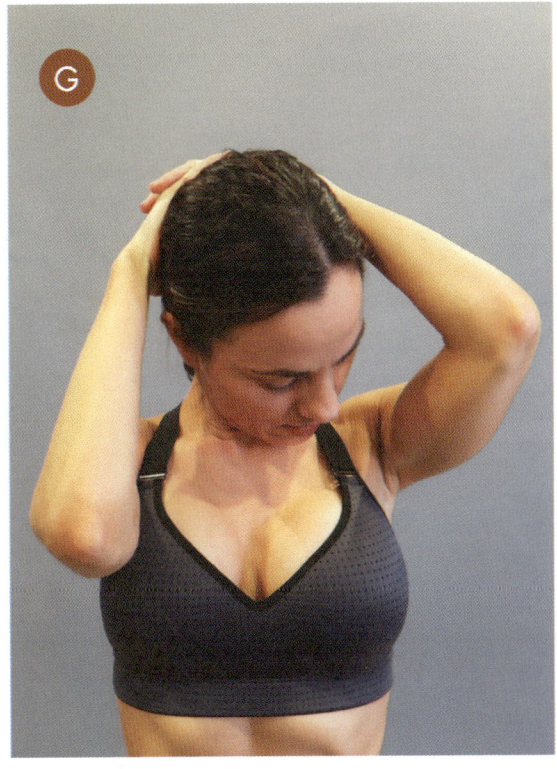

Variations (Image G)

To intensify the stretch on one side, rotate your face toward that side. This combines **flexion** and **rotation**. For example, if you feel tighter in the group of muscles on the left, turn your face a little toward the left. Press a little more on the back of your head with the left hand. This will shift the locus of the stretch to the left side. Hold then relax. When you're done, remove your hands and roll your head gently back towards the centre of your chest.

Flexion B: Atlanto-occipital 'nodding' flexion

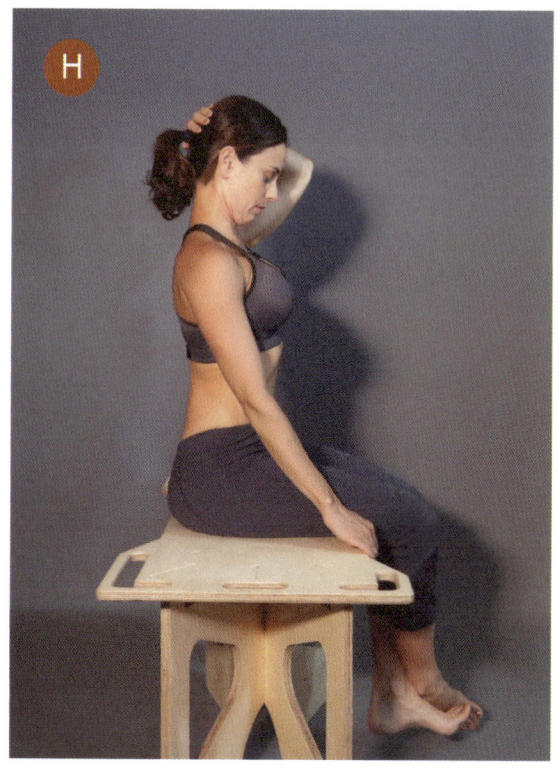

How to stretch (Image H)

Sit up tall, with your weight distributed evenly onto both sit bones. Take your chin toward your neck in a subtle nodding motion and then place your hands gently onto the back of your head as pictured. Take as much of the weight of your hands and arms onto your head as necessary to give you a stretch. As usual, take a deep breath in and relax.

Try not to bend the whole of your neck, just the region that you would use to nod your head. Do not force the issue. Pull gently on your scalp as if you are going to drag the hair from the back of your head onto the top of your head. Tensioning the scalp will increase the stretch.

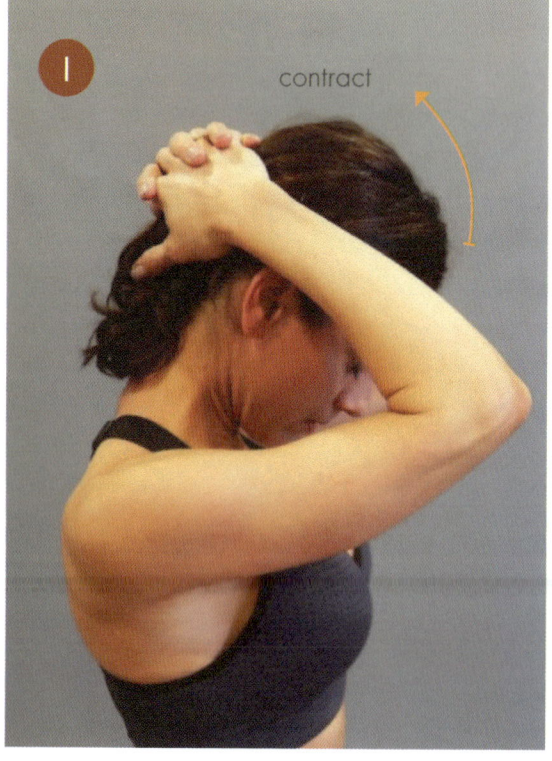

How to contract (Image I)

Lightly lift your chin to the ceiling. Think of this as distinct from pressing the entire head back. Press for 5 seconds with the usual 30% or so of maximum effort.

Flexion B: Atlanto-occipital 'nodding' flexion

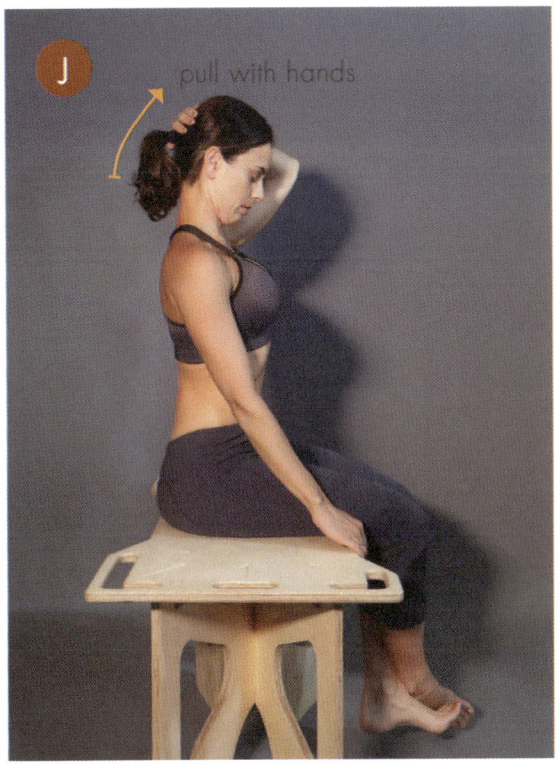

Restretch (Image J)

Take a deep breath in. On the breath out take your chin toward your your neck, as if tucking it back to create a double chin. Use your hands to apply a little more force, and again pull on your scalp. Relax your shoulders and hold for up to ten breaths.

Variations (Image K)

To intensify the stretch on one side, rotate your face toward that side. This combines flexion and rotation. For example, if you feel tighter in the group of muscles on the left, turn your face a little toward the left. Press a little more on the back of your head with the left hand. This will focus the sensation on the sub-occipital muscles at the rear of the neck, where a great deal of tension is stored.

Major Muscles Stretched

- ## Suboccipitals (Deep neck muscles)

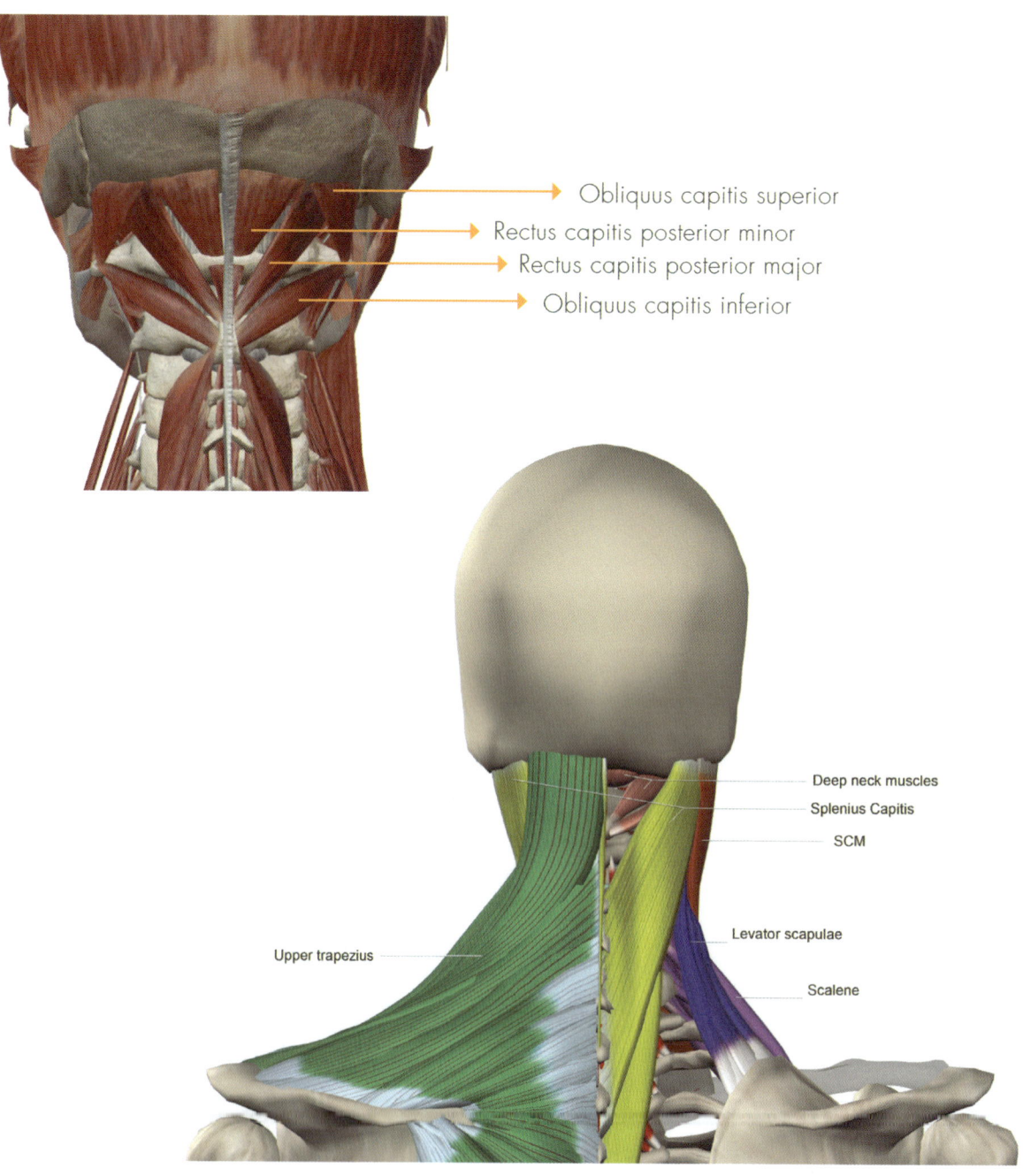

Extension

Background

Pure extension involves taking the head directly backward from the centre position. If performed unsupported, this can be uncomfortable. The discomfort arises from either tightness in the muscles at the front of the neck (and there are many) or from compression of the joints at the back of the neck. If discomfort occurs in either position, try performing extension over some kind of support.

A note of **caution** needs to be sounded here. Strong extension of the neck, particularly with rotation, can result in tearing or compression of the carotid or vertebral arteries. There is little way of telling who may be at risk, but **if you experience dizziness during the exercise you should stop immediately**. (For further information on this subject, read about 'vertebrobasilar insufficiency' below).

This stretch can be valuable for those diagnosed with thoracic outlet syndrome, with symptoms including neck, shoulder and arm pain, and numbness or impaired circulation to the extremities. The stretch focuses on some of the anterior and middle scalene muscles which may be one cause of the syndrome. Those diagnosed with this condition may find this stretch of great benefit.

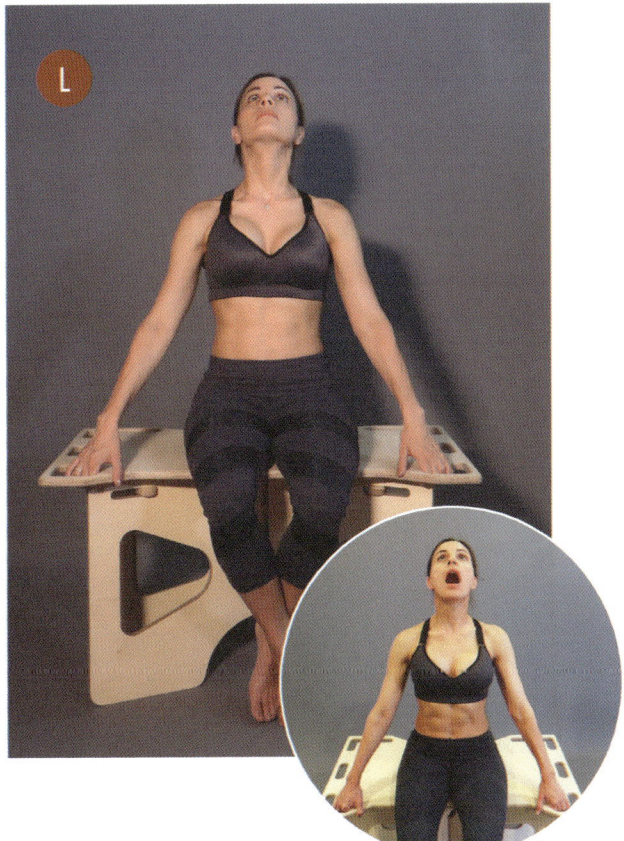

How to stretch (Image L)

Sit comfortably and place your hands into the front slots. Open your mouth and take your head slowly and directly backwards. Close your mouth once your head is as far back as it will comfortably go. Having the mouth open can be gentler at first. As you close your mouth you will feel the stretch increase in the front of your throat. Try to relax and hold for five breaths. While doing so, remain aware of the previous caution about dizziness.

How to contract (Image L)

Make a minimal effort to press your head forward i.e back to neutral for 5 seconds.

Extension

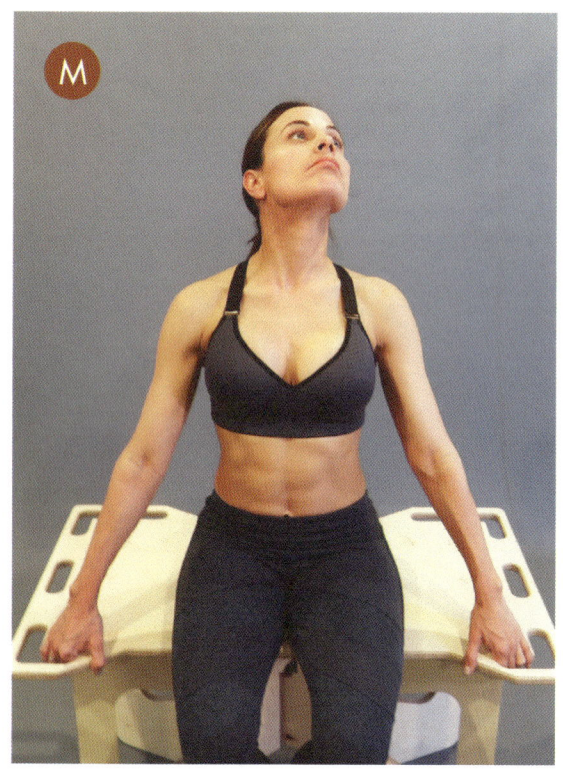

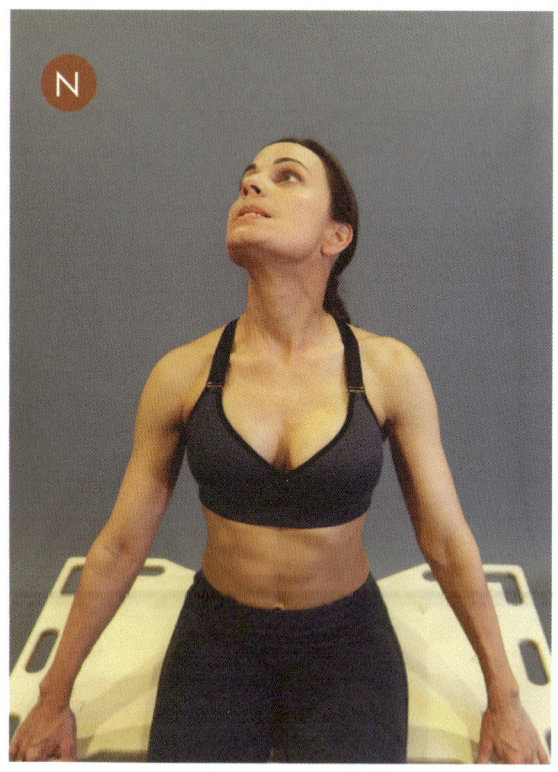

Restretch (Image M & N)

Relax and take your head back a little further. Explore turning your head with tiny movements either left or right. Try lifting your bottom row of teeth above the top row (Image N). This might shift the stretch to directly below your jaw. Play around with it and explore with the slightest of movements. When you have had enough, relax the front arms and roll your head forward gently.

Major Muscles Stretched

- Longus colli
- SCM
- Scalenus anterior
- Longus Capitus

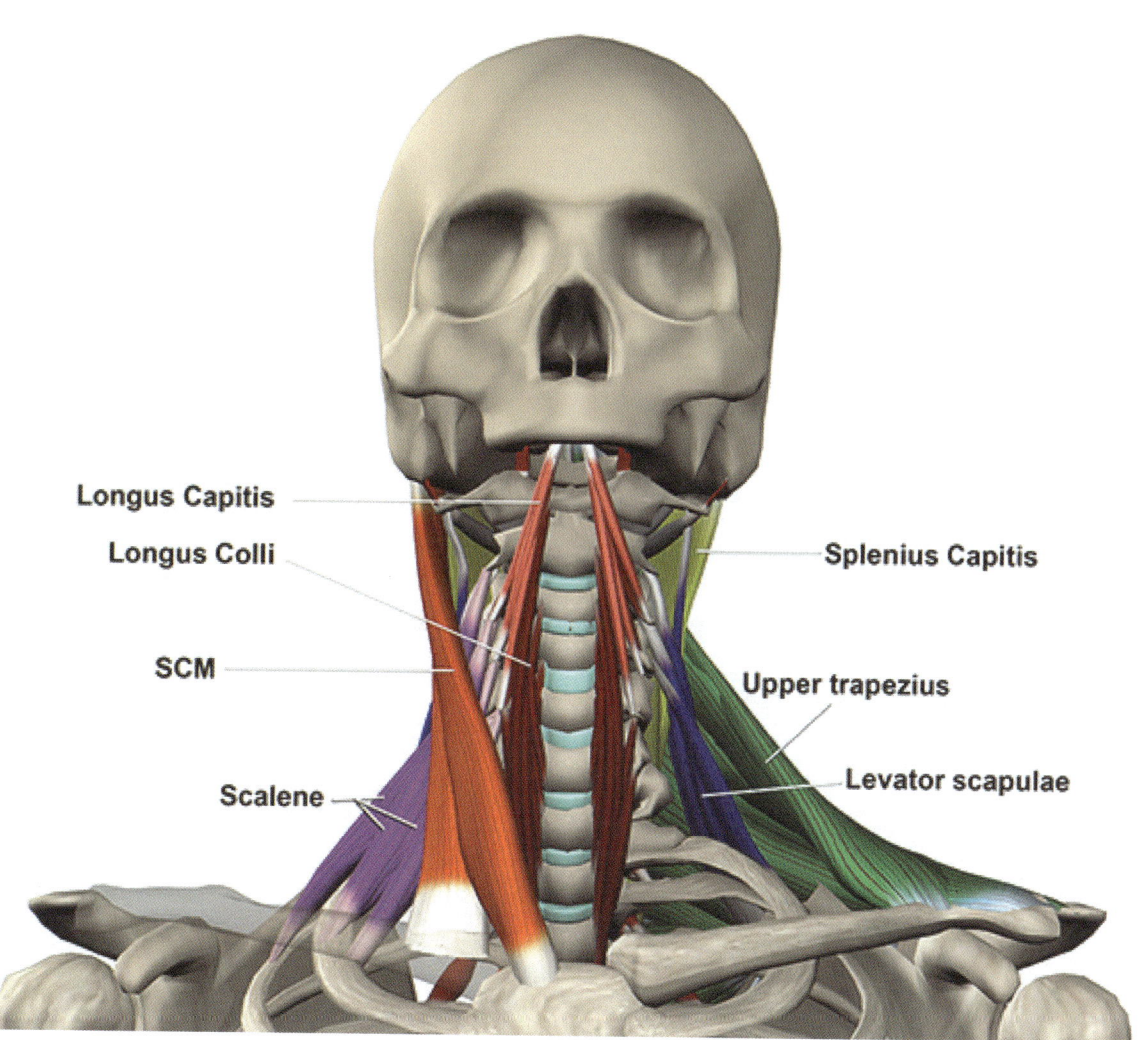

Rotation

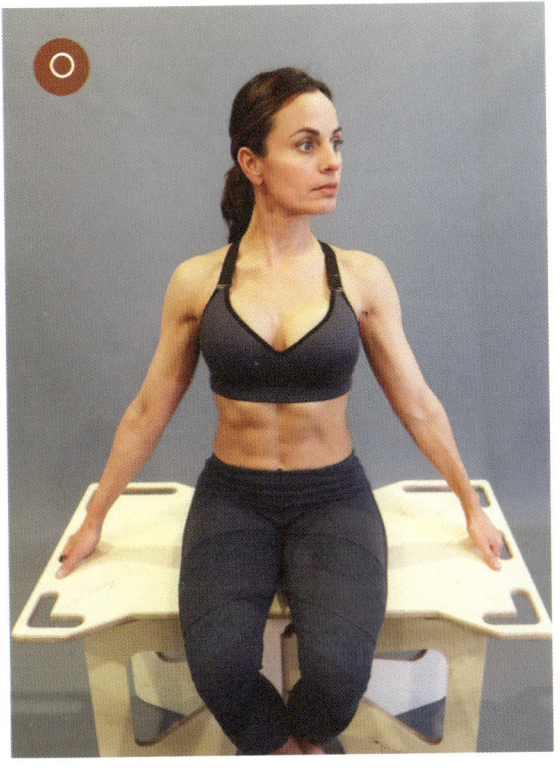

How to stretch (Image O)

Sit as pictured and with your hands in the slots. Turn your face/head to one side. Take it as far as is comfortable. Hold the position for five breaths.

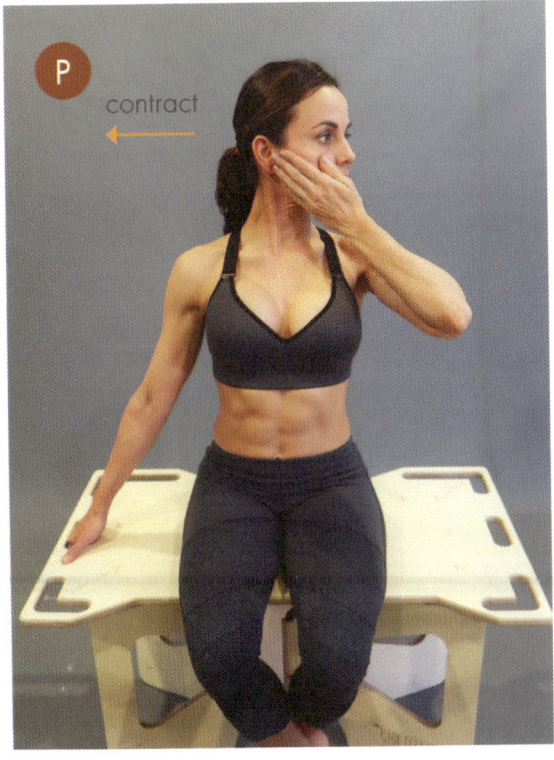

How to contract (Image P)

Reach up with the hand on the same side that you are turning to and place it on your cheek. For example, if you are turning to the left, use your left hand and place it onto your right cheek. Gently, press your head back toward the center position, or into your hand. Either cue will suffice. Prevent any movement of your head occurring with your hand. Press for 5 seconds.

Rotation

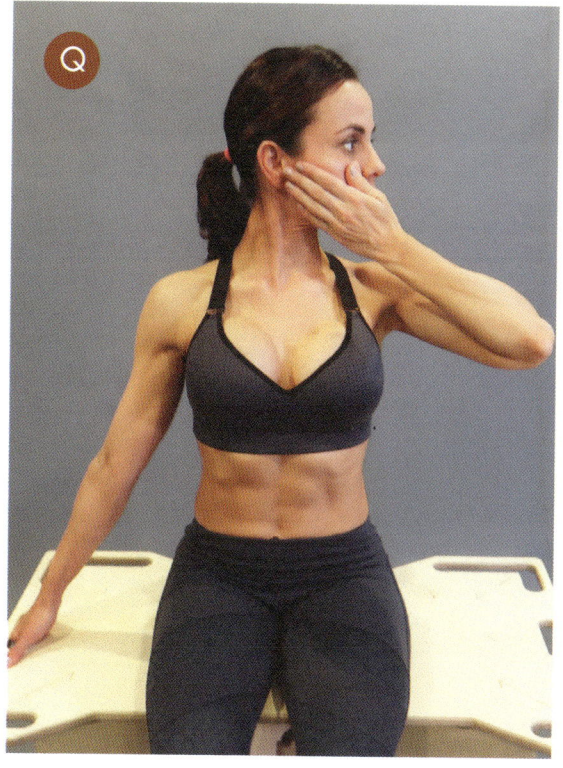

Restretch (Image Q)

Relax and on a breath out, turn your face further away from the center. See if you can look over the shoulder. You can use your hand to press your head lightly to increase the rotation. Hold for the usual period of 10 to 15 breaths.

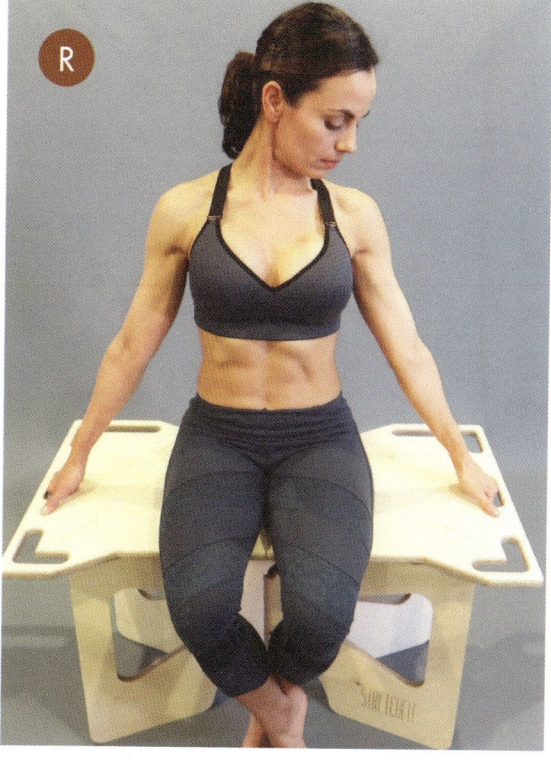

Variation (Image R)

Combining rotation with slight flexion may bring about different sensation. Once in the rotated position, try a minute nod of the head. If it does change the locus of the stretch, hold for 5 to 10 breaths.

Major Muscles Stretched

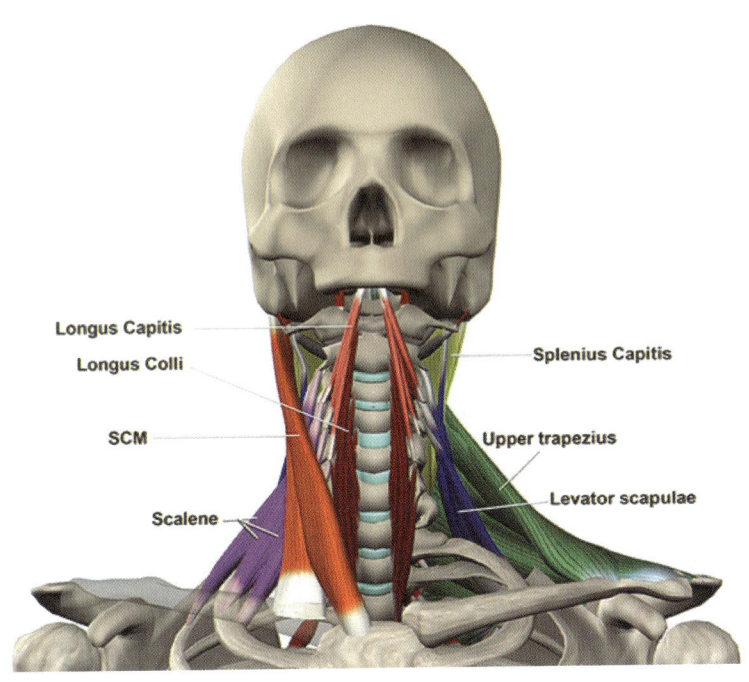

- SCM
- Splenius
- Levator scapulae
- Upper trapezius

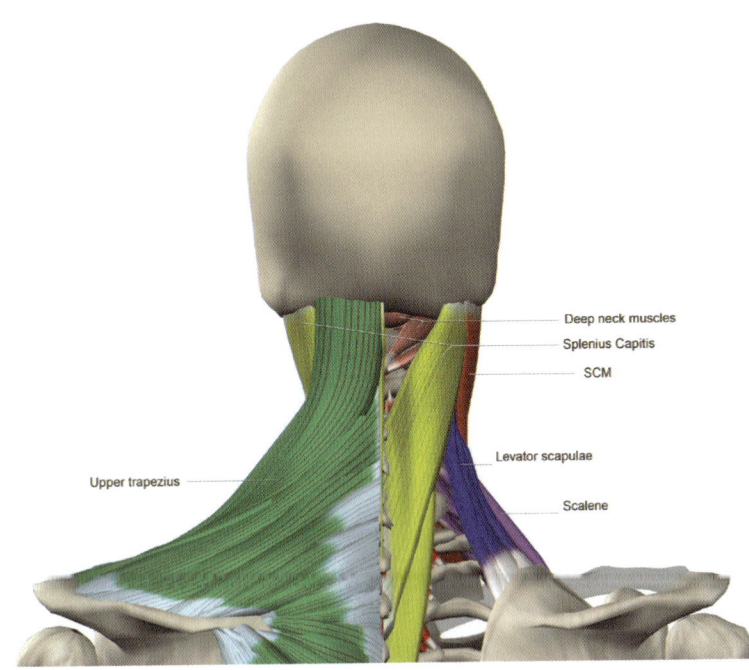

- Deep neck muscles
- Upper trapezius
- Levator scapulae

Vertebrobasilar insufficiency

Mechanical forces acting upon the neck at any age can cause VBI by exacerbating arterial insufficiency or outright occluding one or both vertebrobasilar arteries.

Internal forces include those caused by turning the head to an extreme angle to the side, especially with the neck extended. The person can create this condition while practicing yoga, driving a vehicle in reverse, shooting a bow and arrow, bird watching, or stargazing. External forces include those caused by sports or other physical contact.

VBI was first reported in the early 1990s when an American neurologist identified five patients who suffered strokes as a result of prolonged distortion of their necks from sitting at salon wash basins.

In 1997 medical journal The Lancet published a report by two British doctors about a 42-year-old woman who suffered a stroke after having her hair washed.

The experts said the stroke was due to "dissection of her right internal carotid artery. Her head had been extended backwards for about five minutes while being washed and after the treatment she felt numb and suffered slurred speech."

The doctors recommended that hairdressers use a cushion and that the neck is not overextended. As a result of this recommendation there have been several sink cushions developed including Nekeze, Hairtools Basin Neck Cushion and the Soft n Style cushion. Trainee Hairdressers are also being taught to make sure that their clients are comfortable. Several recent studies of the causes of strokes have identified how salon washing basins exert stress on the neck, causing the carotid or vertebral arteries to tear.

David Bateman, a consultant neurologist at Cumberland Infirmary, said that "salon hairwashing was an identifiable, if small, risk factor for people predisposed to arterial damage. If your neck is stretched and it kinks for a long time, as happens during hairwashing, you stretch the arteries and if you are unlucky you can tear them," he added "Once you have got that tear in the lining, blood starts flowing between layers of tissue and that can cause blood clots to start building up, leading to a stroke."

Dr Bateman went onto say "stroke cases from neck overextension appeared only in people particularly vulnerable to arterial tears, although there was little way of telling who might be at risk. Other factors that contribute to strokes include high blood pressure, diabetes, smoking and raised cholesterol."

Other such triggers, which normally require ten minutes of neck overextension, include fairground rides, dentists' chairs, sit-up exercises and yoga. Another cause, known as Golden Gate Bridge Syndrome, is prompted by excessive strain of looking up.

Additional Variations

The Combination Variation

Background

This stretch combines cervical flexion with lateral flexion and rotation. It is similar to a movement explored above but this time the hand is placed in the rear slot. By depressing the scapula this tends to focus the stretch in the large posterior muscles of the neck including the splenius, levator scapula and upper trapezius muscles.

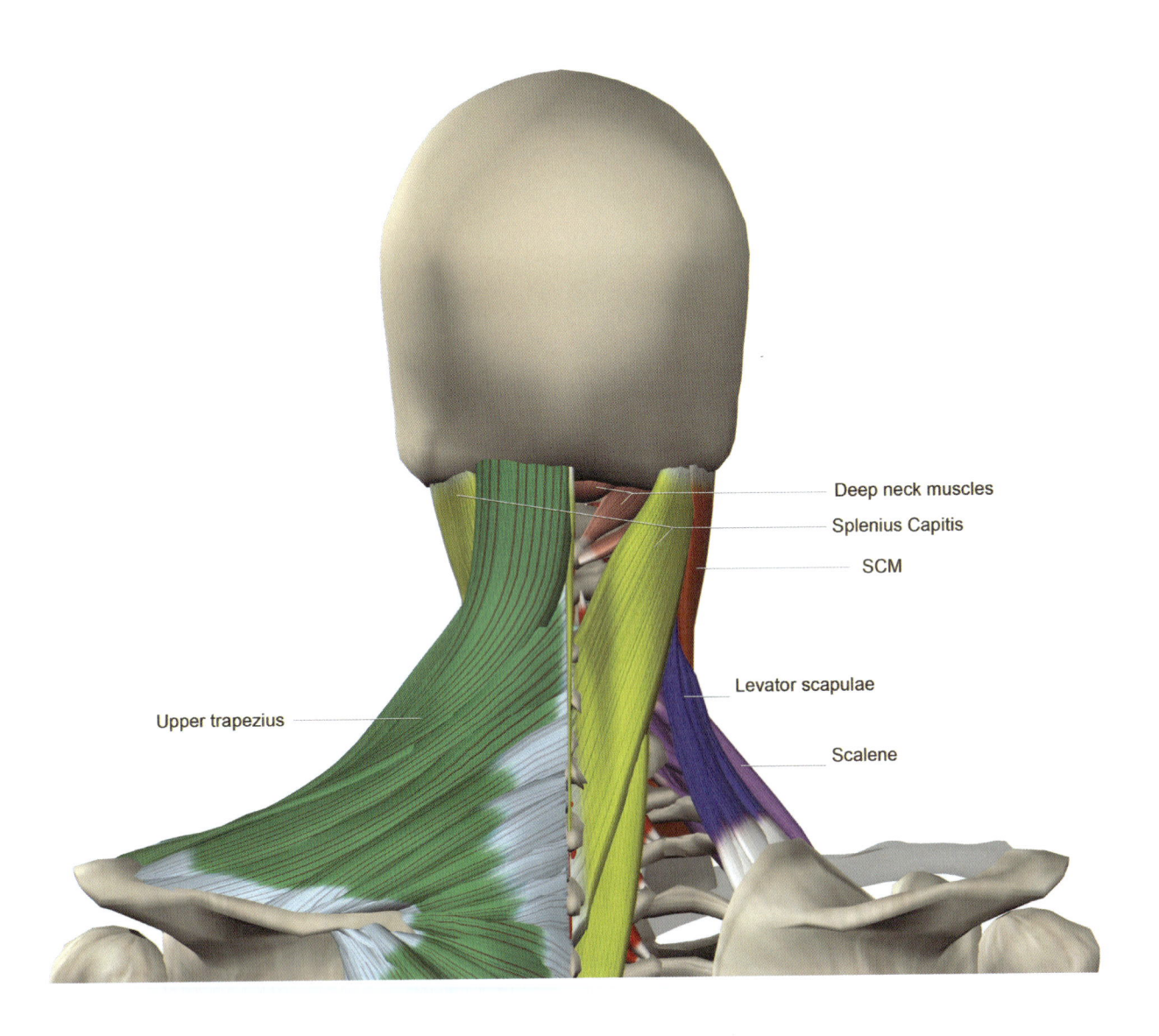

The Combination Variation

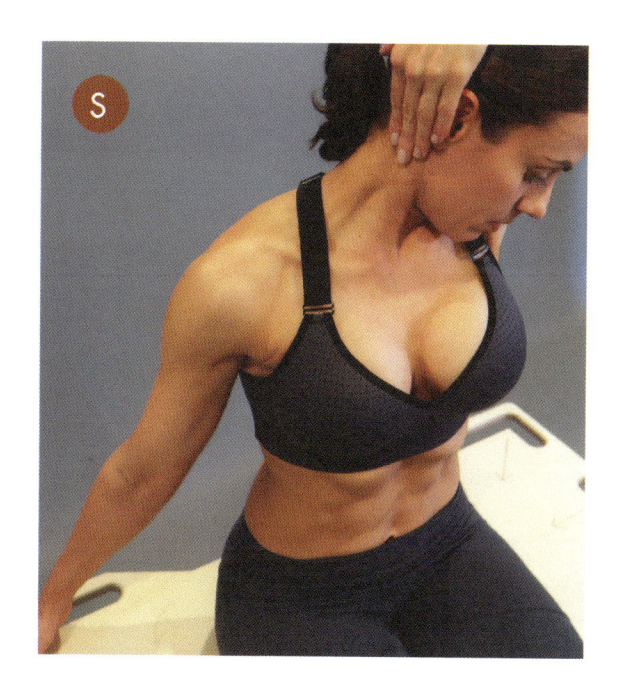

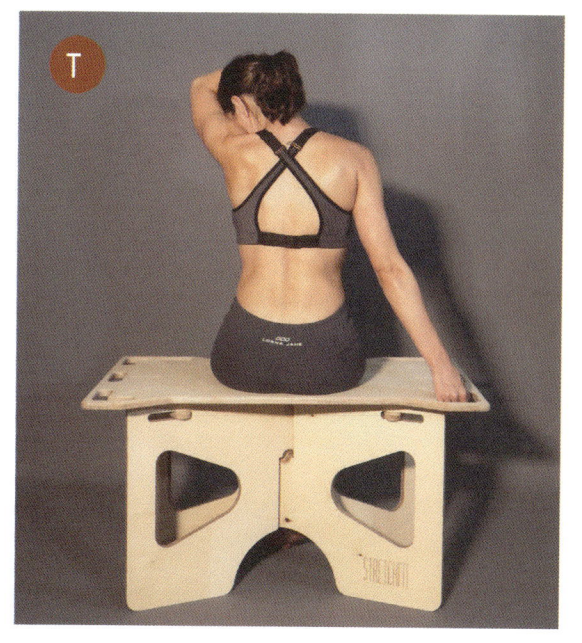

How to stretch (Image S)

Sit in the center of the chair and restrain the shoulder by reaching one hand behind into the rear slot. Lean directly away from the rear/restraining hand. If you find that your sit bone is lifting, adjust your sitting position so that you begin by being seated a bit further from the rear slot, toward the front of the seat. Take your chin down toward your chest and then take your head across toward the opposite armpit. Reach the free arm up and place it over your head so that your fingers rest just behind your ear.

How to contract (Image S & T)

Press your head lightly back into your hand, toward the rear hand that is in the slot.

Restretch

Take a breath in and on a breath out, lean further away from the rear hand. Use the hand on your head to press or pull gently on your scalp. You can explore turning your head slowly toward your armpit further and see how it feels. Also, try turning your face away from the armpit. No position is wrong. As you have discovered, there are dozens of muscles in the region and your work is to locate the tight ones. Make all movements very slowly with great care and attention. If you locate a tight spot, hold the position. To finish, roll your chin toward your chest and back to the center. As always repeat on the other side.

Flexion of the entire spine

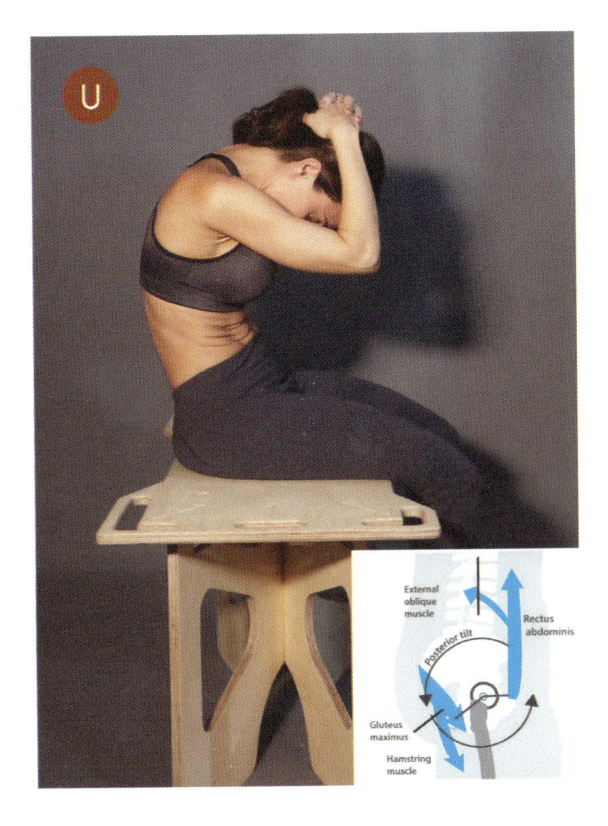

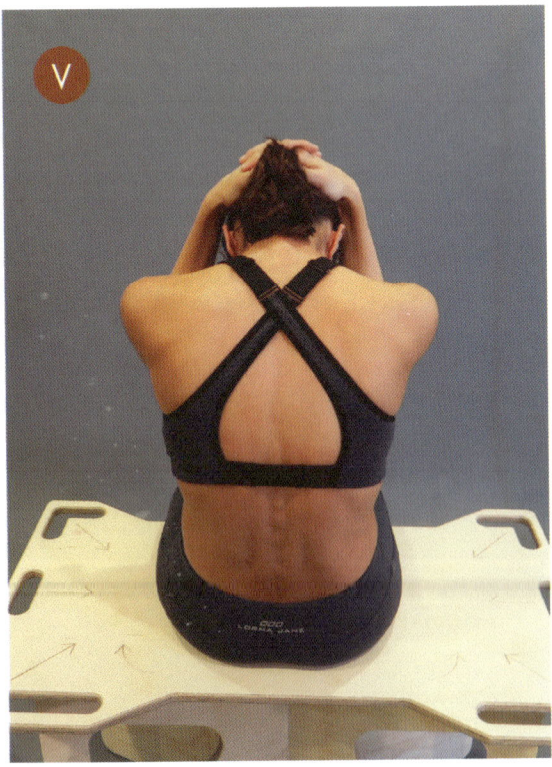

How to stretch (Image U and V)

This stretch moves the experience from just the neck down the entire posterior aspect of the trunk. Dozens of muscles occupy the region and it is common for a variety of stretches to be found by exploring slight changes in position.

To begin, center yourself on the seat and place both hands lightly onto the back of your head (not the top). Relax your shoulders, take your chin to your chest and and take as much of the weight of your arms as is comfortable.

Next, allow your pelvis to roll backwards and your head to drop toward your lap. Note that this is a slump position and should not require any effort at all. If you are leaning backwards, you are not relaxed. You head should fall toward your lap. Find your balance point that is a "no effort required" position.

Relax your elbows and shoulders as the weight of your head and your arms flexes your trunk. Hold for 5 deep breaths.

As the entire spine is flexed the muscles that run parallel to the spinal column itself, called the erector spinae are stretched.

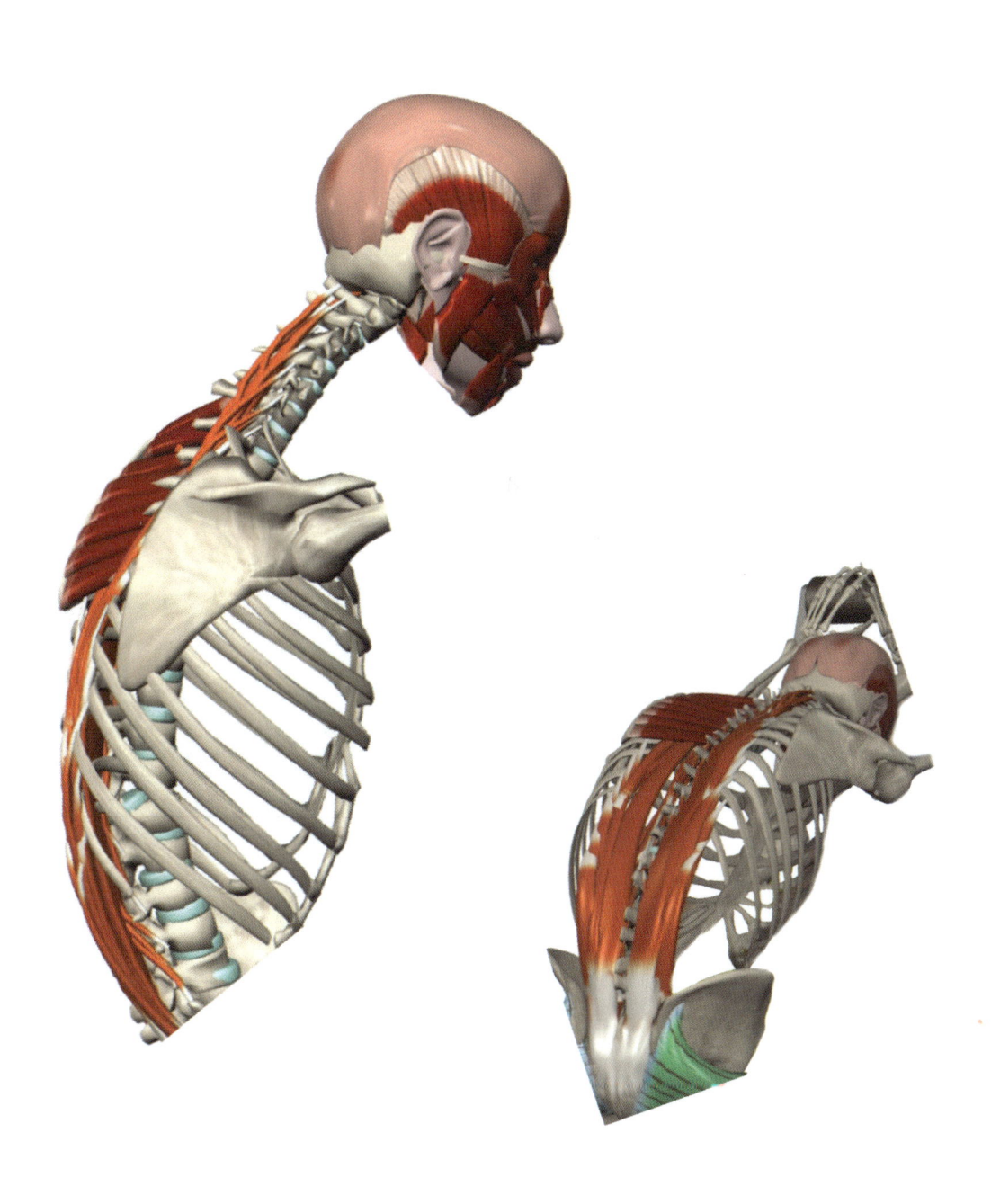

Flexion of the entire spine

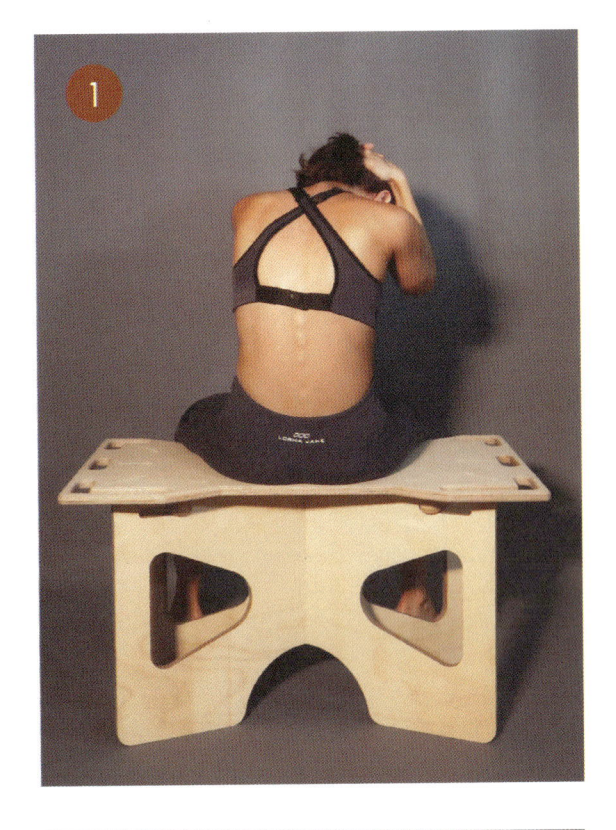

Variation One

Slowly rotate your shoulders so that your thigh is between your elbows. If you have turned to the right as in the image 1, the stretch will likely increase down the left side of the spine. You can play around with subtle changes in the degree of rotation of your spine and your neck.

Hold for at least five breaths and repeat on the other side.

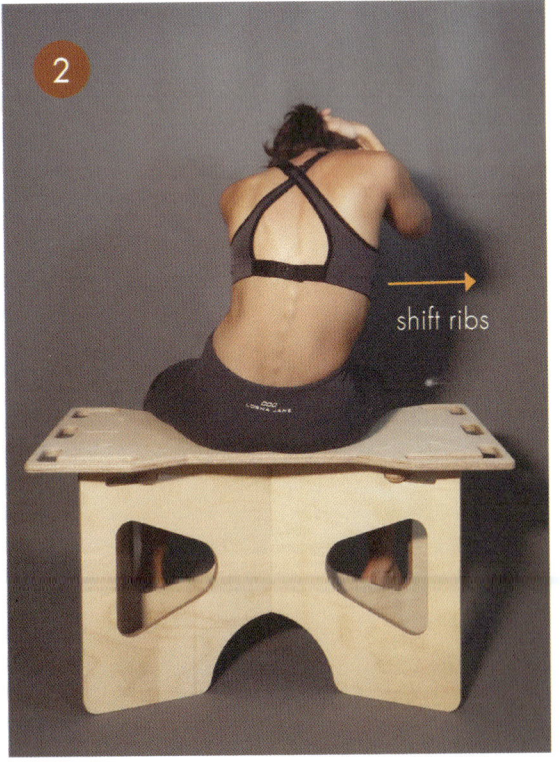

Variation Two

In addition to the rotation above, shift your ribcage across also. Shift it toward the side you are rotating toward. For example, right side rotation, right side rib shift. See image 2. This might diminish the sensation a bit on the left side of the spine, but increase them on the right, in particular between the shoulder blade and the spine.

Explore things and breathe deeply. Don't lose your slump as you attempt these variations. As above, no position is wrong if done with care and gentle curiosity.

Flexion of the entire spine

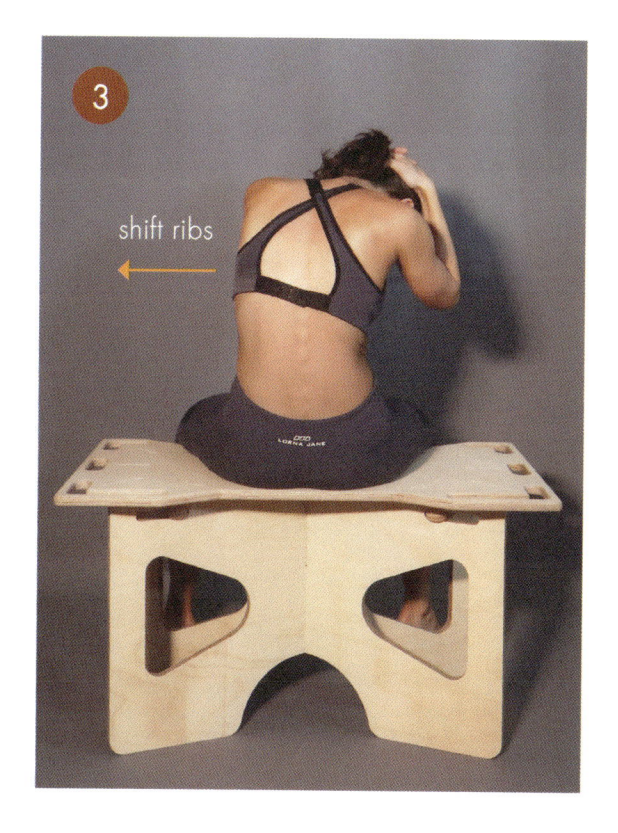

shift ribs

Variation Three

Shift your ribcage way from the side that you are rotating toward. i.e rotation to the right with rib cage shift to the left. See image 3.

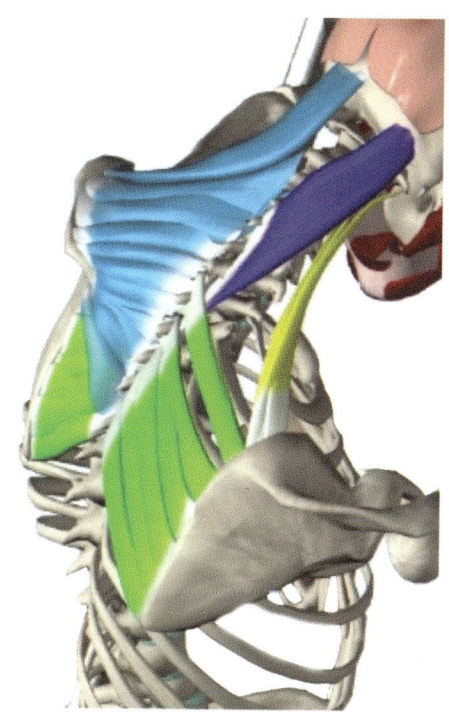

Some of the obliquely oriented muscles that work on the scapula like the trapezius, rhomboids and levator scapula will stretch especially with the variations to this stretch.

- Trapezius
- Rhomboids
- Levator scapulae

Text Neck   43

Seated rotation of the entire spine

Background

Because of the shape and configuration of the lumbar vertebrae, it is only able to rotate around 5 degrees in either direction. Almost all the rotation of the spine in this stretch is therefore in the thoracic and cervical spine. Although a large number of muscles are stretched during this movement, in particular the oblique abdominal muscles, it often does not feel like other stretches.

The sensation that you feel is often the rotation of the joints of the spine rather than the stretching of muscles. This does not mean you are doing it wrongly, or that you are not benefitting. In fact, spinal rotation is essential for the health of the joints and their disks. To exaggerate the stretch in the obliques, breath as deeply as you can.

Deep breathing will expand the muscles in the region. As the diaphragm descends, it is the equivalent of inflating the entire region from within. This balloons out the region and stretches the overlying muscles.

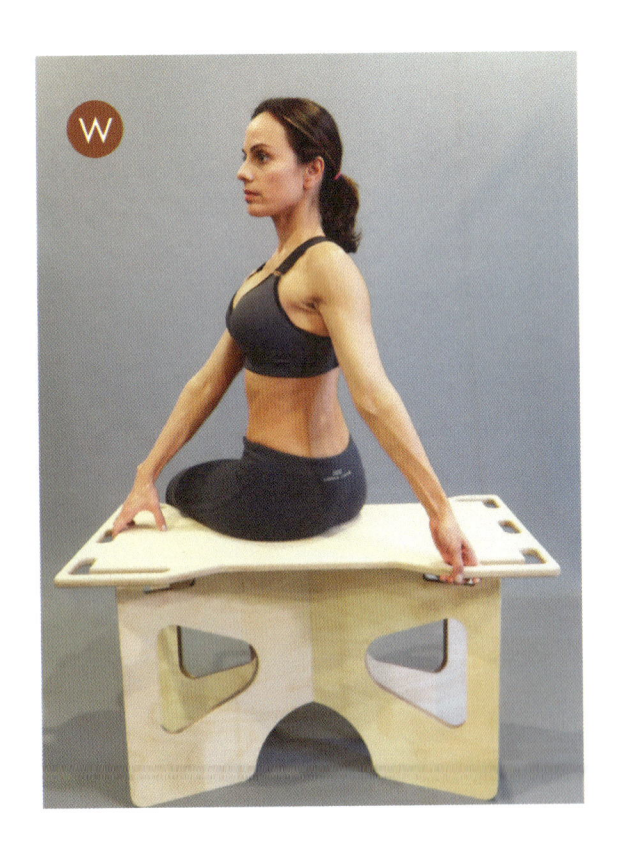

How to stretch (Image W)

Sit as pictured with your legs against one side of the seat. This will anchor the base of your spine inside the pelvic bones. Lift your chest and rotate your trunk to away from your legs.

Place your hands inside any slots and use them to assist with your rotation. Be sure to sit upright and keep your chest lifted. Hold for five deep breaths.

Seated rotation of the entire spine

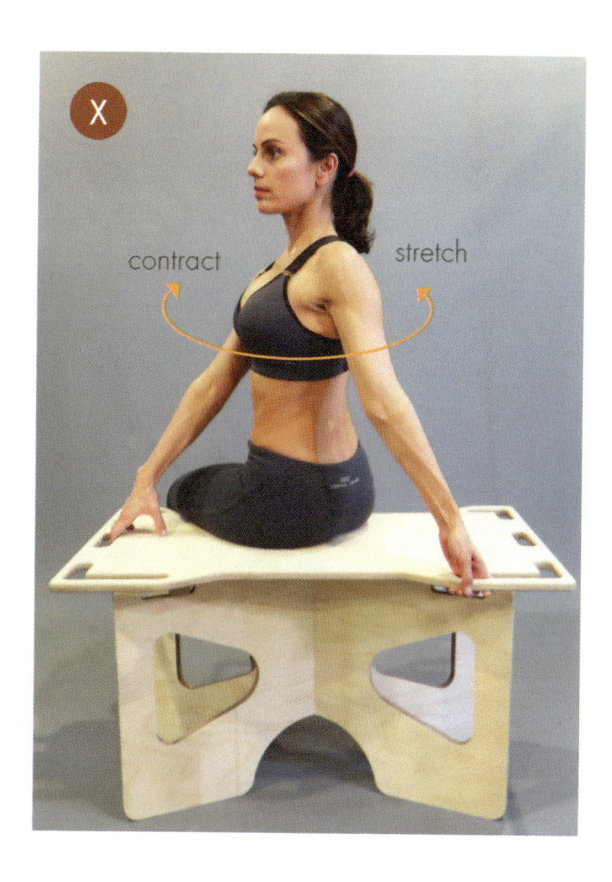

How to Contract (Image X)

With only a little force, try to turn your chest and shoulders back toward the starting position. Prevent any movement with your arms. Contract for 5 seconds.

How to restretch

Take a breath in and on a breath out, use your arms to take you into further rotation. Turn your head also for maximum stretch in the neck. Check your posture and lift your chest.

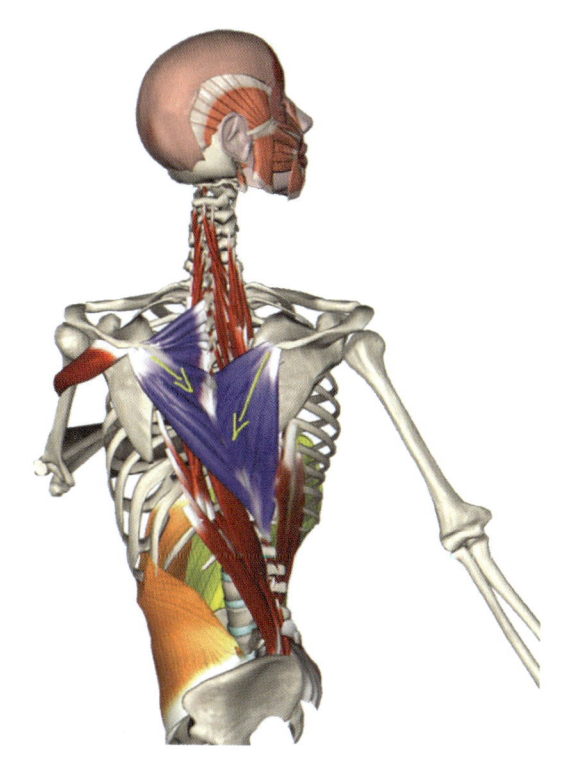

Draw your shoulders blades back and down to assist in opening the chest and maintaining a good upright position.

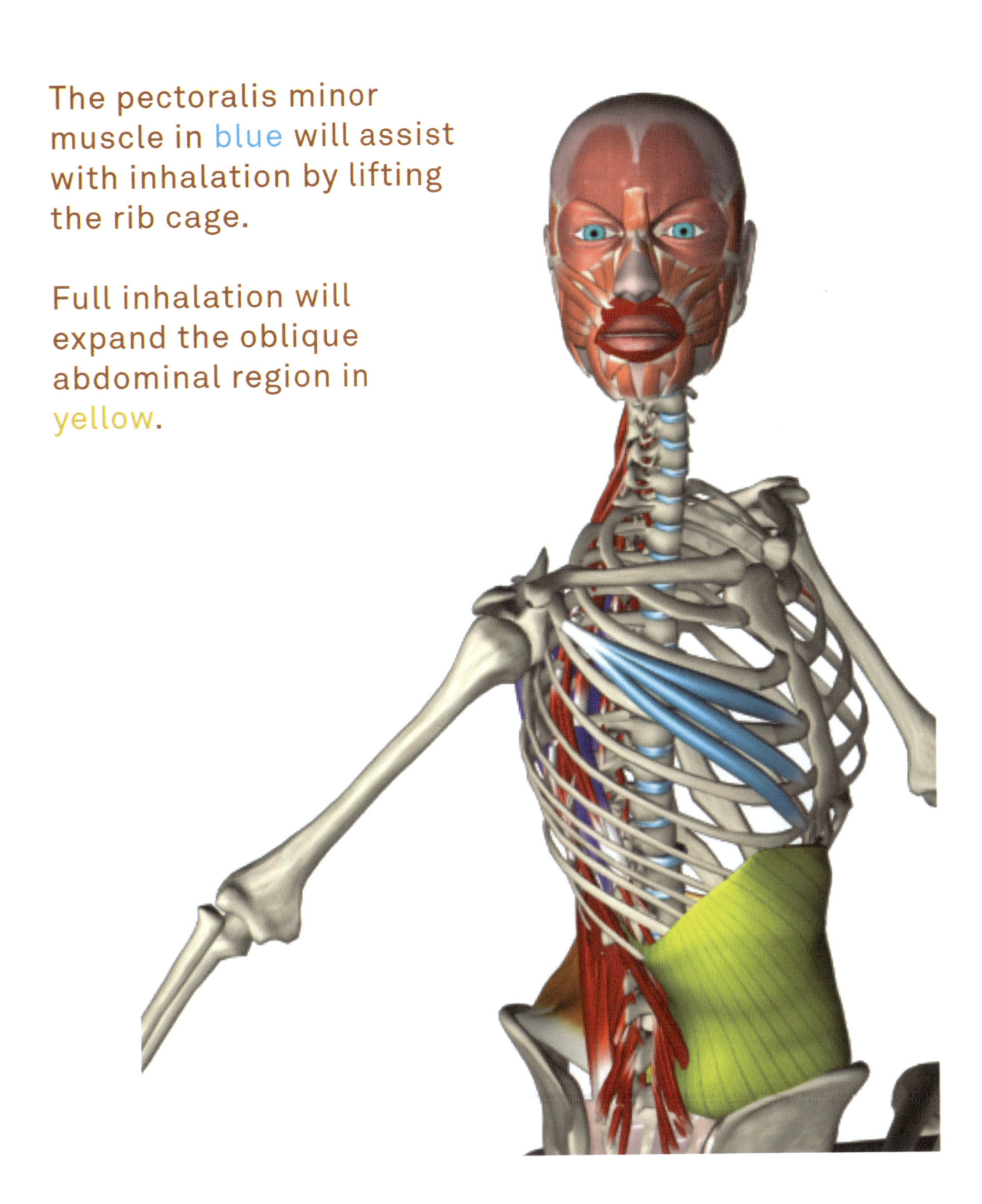

The pectoralis minor muscle in blue will assist with inhalation by lifting the rib cage.

Full inhalation will expand the oblique abdominal region in yellow.

46 Text Neck

Thoracic extension

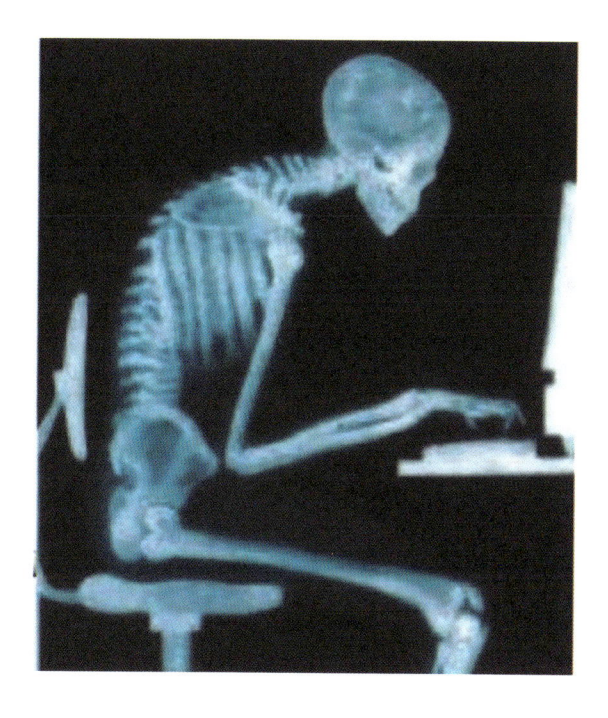

Background

The image to the left, although slightly exaggerated, demonstrates the pronounced curvature in the upper thoracic spine that often accompanies text neck. Muscle and joint pain in the region as well as shoulder dysfunction often develop as a result. The length of the spinous processes in the thoracic region does not permit it to bend backwards like the cervical and lumbar region. However, the joints can be mobilised, and the surrounding muscles stretched to permit the upper back to reverse its usual curve and to flatten. In the stretch below, we are trying to flatten the thoracic spine. It may not feel like a strong muscular stretch but unless you have pain deep in the shoulder joint (an impingement sign) persevere.

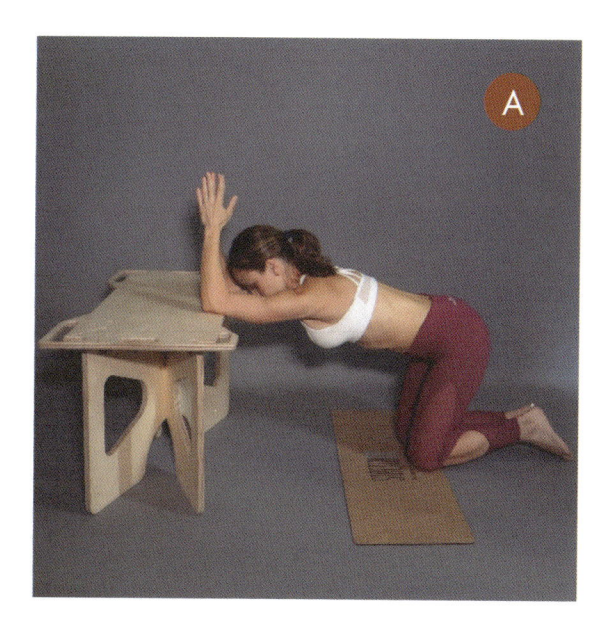

How to stretch (Image A & B)

Place your arms on the neck deck or chair, just above your elbows.

Position your knees below your hips.

Lower your chest toward the floor.

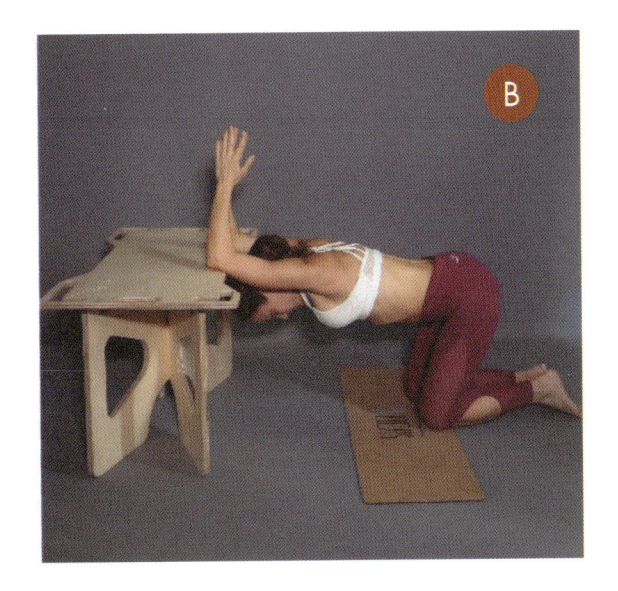

How to contract (Image B)

Press your elbows down into the deck, without any observable movement.

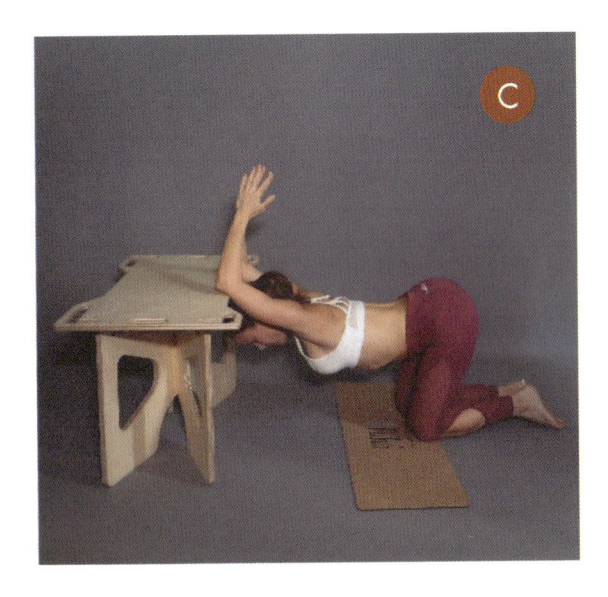

How to restretch (Image C)

Lower your chest further towards the floor.

Quick Reference Guide

Neck Flexion

How to stretch (Photo A)
- Tuck chin towards neck or chest.

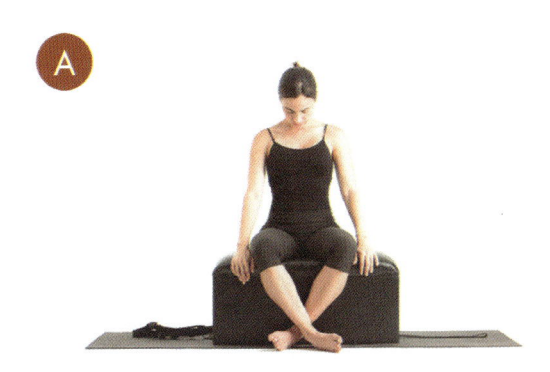

How to Contract (Photo B)
- Place hands onto back of head
- Take as much weight onto head as is comfortable
- Press head back into hands

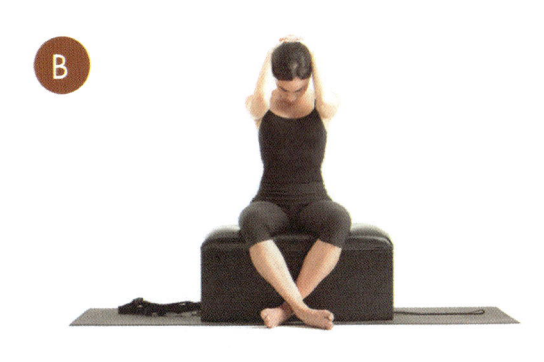

How to Restretch (Photo C)
- Take chin further to neck

Variation (Photo C)
- Turn face towards both armpits
- If turning to right, press with right hand onto head then repeat on other side

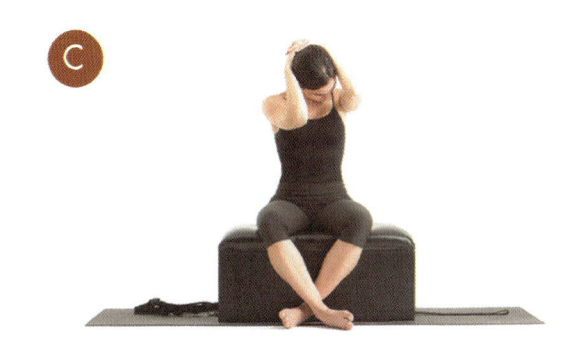

Major Muscles Stretched
- Suboccipitals
- Upper trapezius
- Splenius

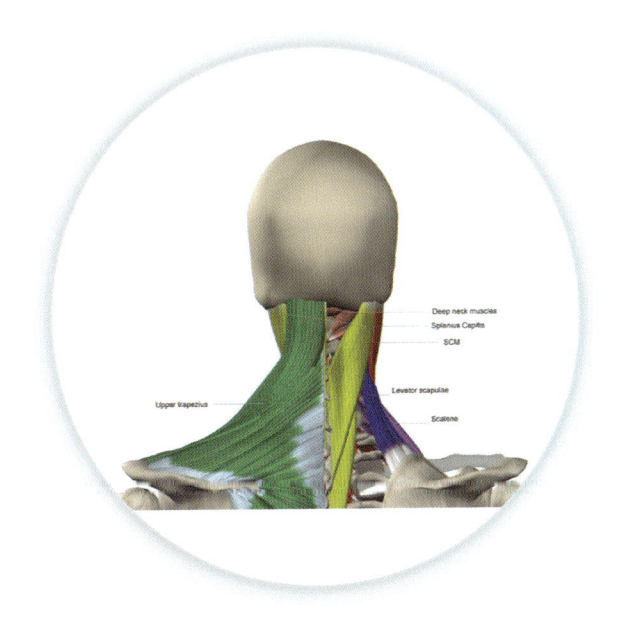

50 Text Neck

The Combination Variation

How to stretch (Photo A, B & C)
- Place hand behind hip in slot
- Relax shoulders and lean away from hand
- Take chin towards chest and turn face to one shoulder
- Reach opposite hand and place it over head
- Rest head onto arm and shoulder

How to Contract (Photo C)
- Press head back towards rear arm/hand

How to Restretch (Photo C)
- Take chin further to chest and turn face further to armpit

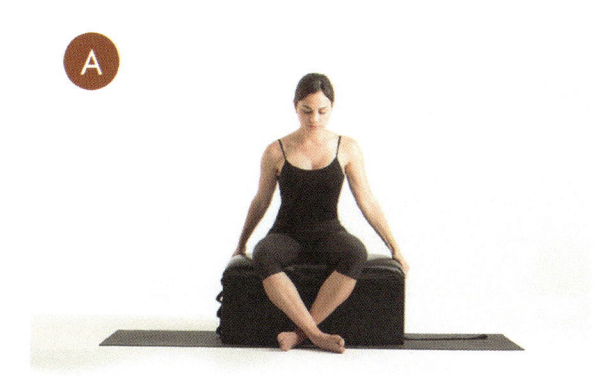

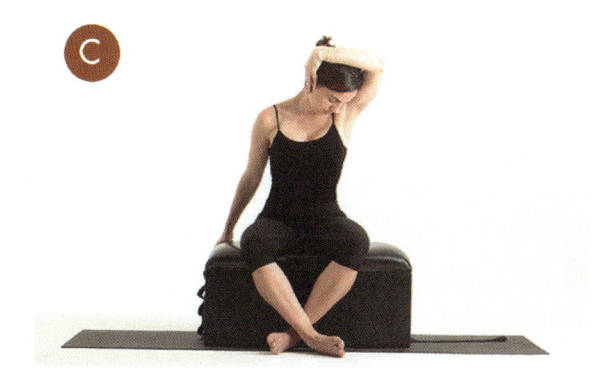

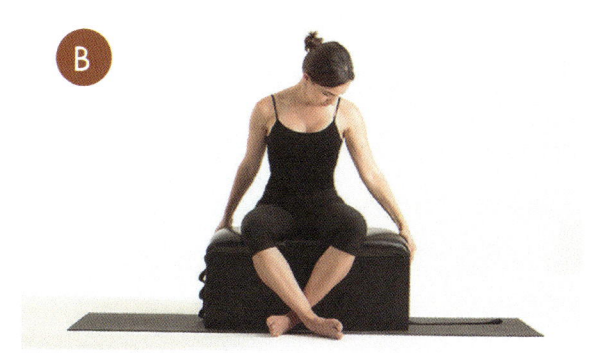

Major Muscles Stretched
- Levator scapula
- Upper trapezius

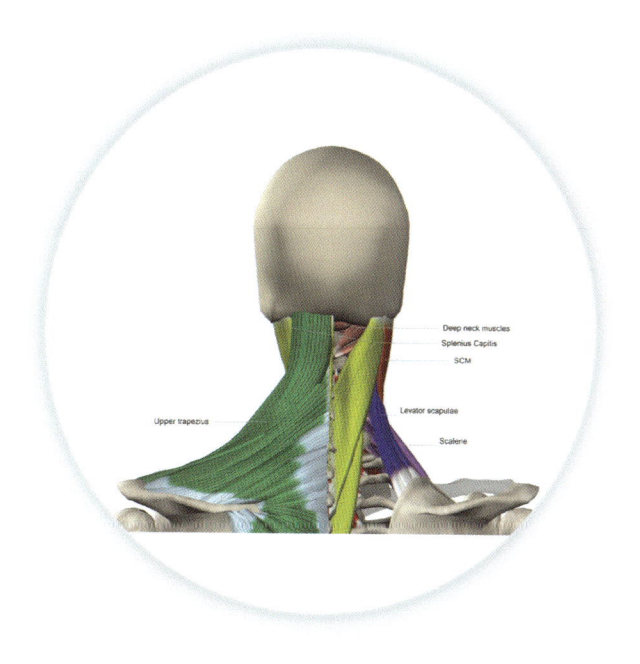

Neck Lateral Flexion

How to stretch (Photo A & B)
- Place arm alongside hip, in line with shoulder
- Insert hand into slot
- Lean away from arm and take head towards opposite shoulder
- Reach opposite arm over head
- Rest head onto opposite arm or shoulder

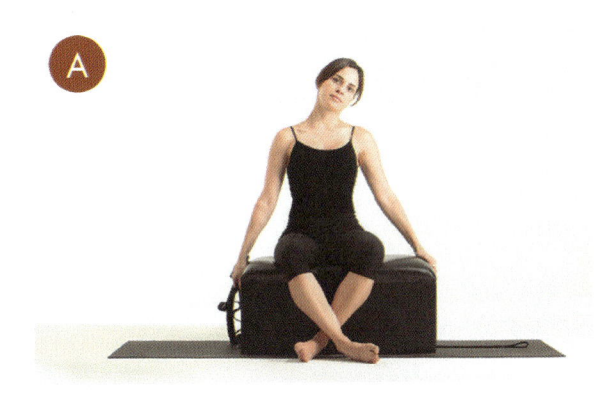

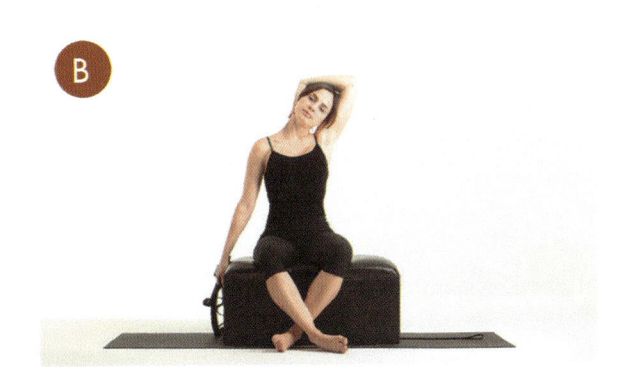

How to Restretch (Photo C)
- Take head further towards opposite shoulder
- Rest head onto shoulder/arm
- Use finger to pull lightly on head
- Turn face towards armpit

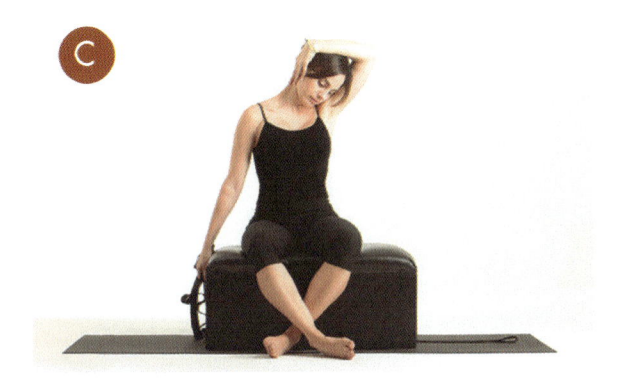

How to Contract (Photo B)
- Press head back towards start position/centre

Major Muscles Stretched
- Scalenus medius and posterior
- Upper trapezius

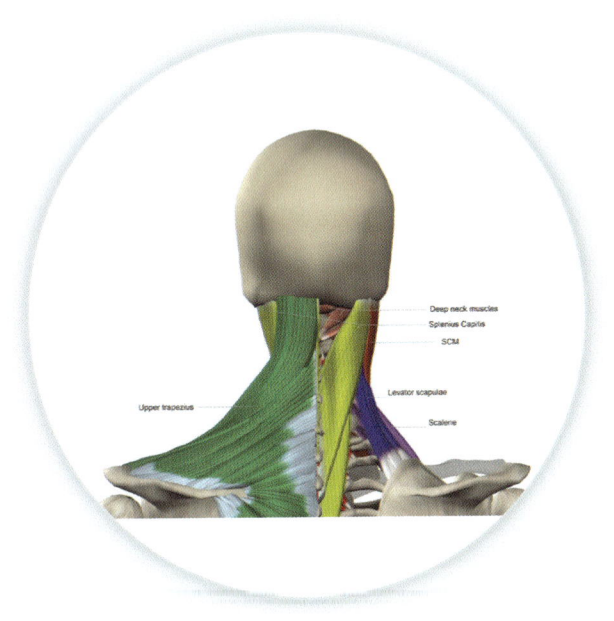

52   Text Neck

Neck Rotation

How to stretch (Photo A & B)
- Turn face towards shoulder
- Prevent shoulders from moving by placing hands into rear slots.
- Place hand onto side of face. If turning to left, use left hand

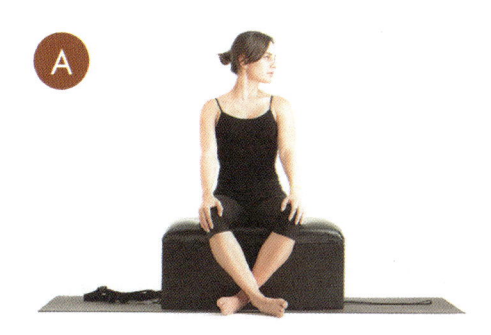

Major Muscles Stretched
- SCM
- Splenius
- Levator scapulae

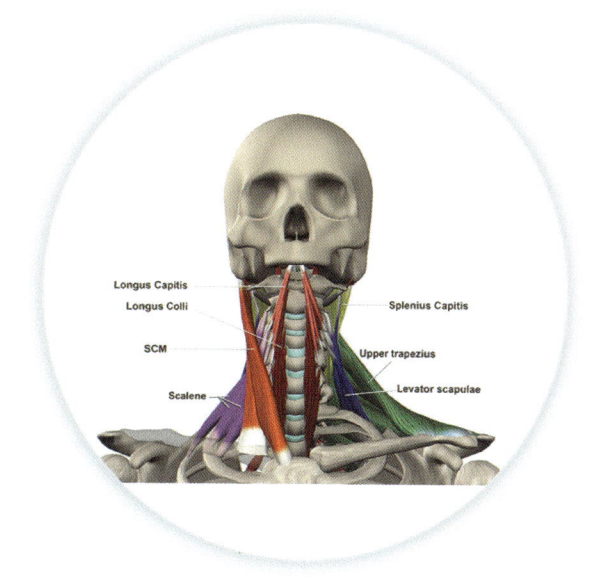

A

How to Contract (Photo B)
- Press head back towards centre/hand

How to Restretch (Photo B & C)
- Turn face further from centre

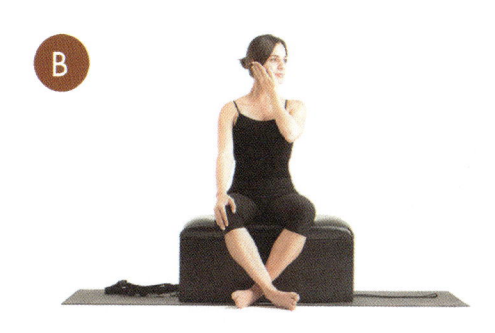

Deep neck muscles
- Upper trapezius
- Levator scapulae

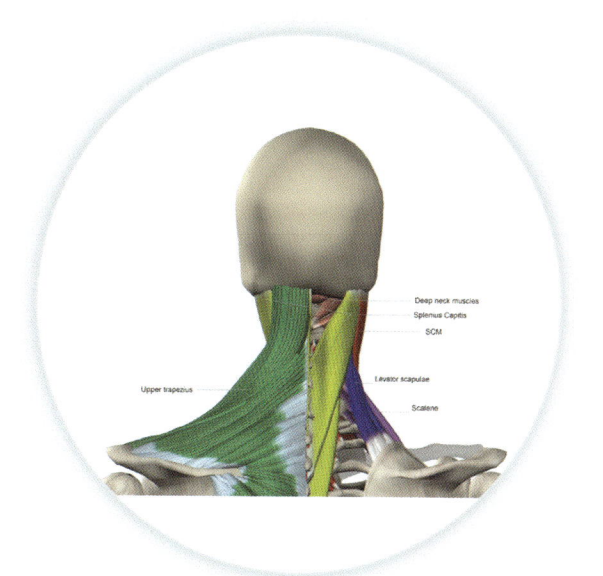

B

Variation (Photo C)
- Turn face and nod head

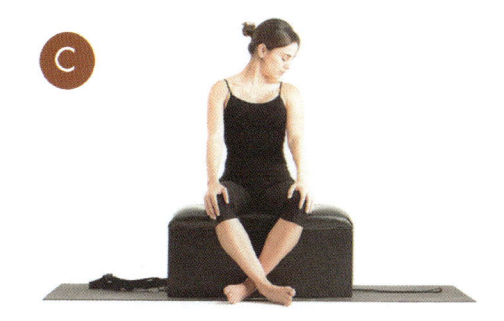

C

Text Neck 53

Neck Extension and Rotation

How to stretch (Photo A & B)
- Place hands into front slots
- Take head backwards with mouth open and then slowly close teeth
- Turn face to one side so that it lines up with one of your hands

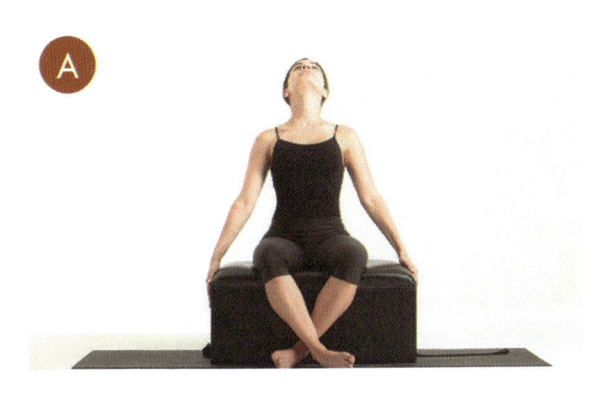

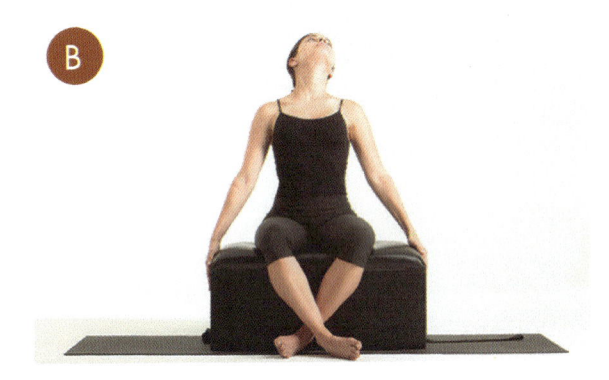

Variation (Photo B & C)
- Turn face fractionally to one side and then the other
- Place bottom row of teeth above top row (undershot bite pattern)

CAUTION: IF YOU EXPERIENCE DIZZINESS DURING THIS STRETCH STOP IMMEDIATELY

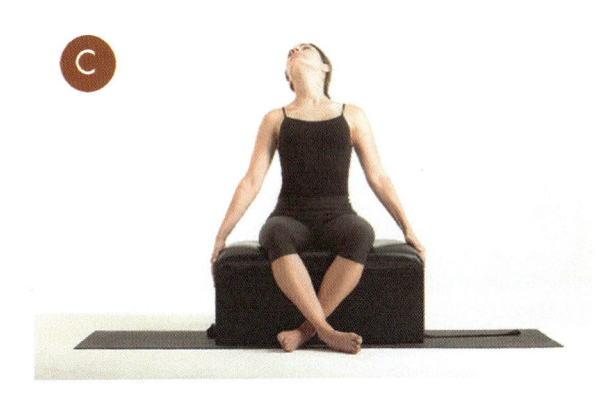

Major Muscles Stretched
- Longus colli
- SCM
- Scalenus anterior

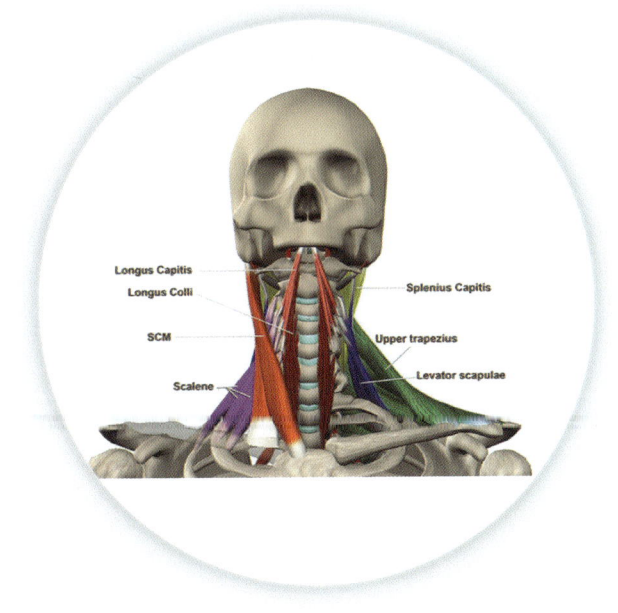

54 Text Neck

Jaw Extension

How to stretch (Photo A & B)

- Wash hands
- Sit in neutral position
- Open mouth and place two or three fingers on bottom front teeth
- Pull down on teeth to open mouth wider
- Clasp side of box for balance

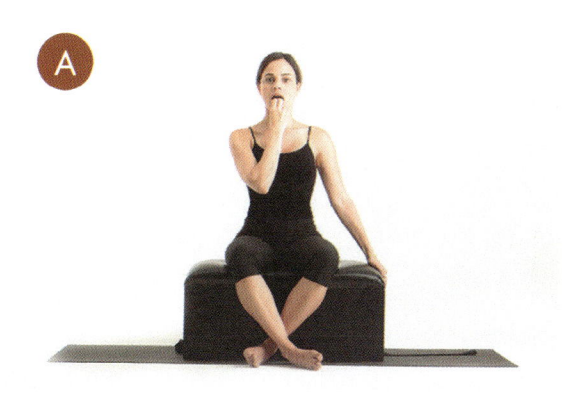

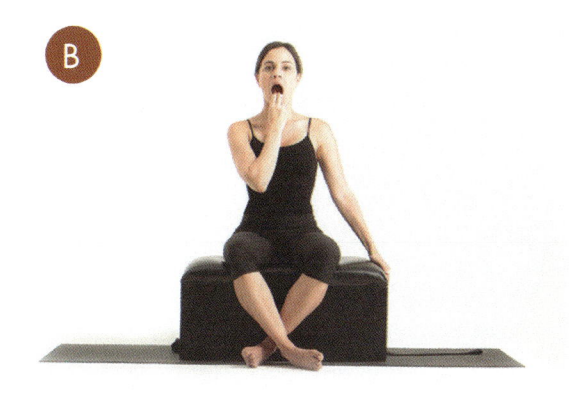

How to Restretch (Photo C & D)

- Pull down further onto jaw and open mouth wider

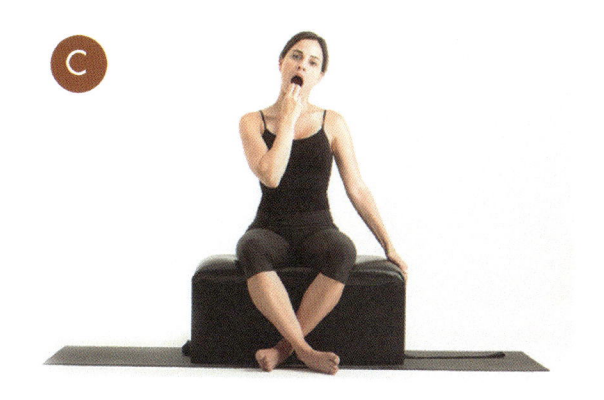

Variation (Photo D)

- Pull down on jaw while tilting head left and right

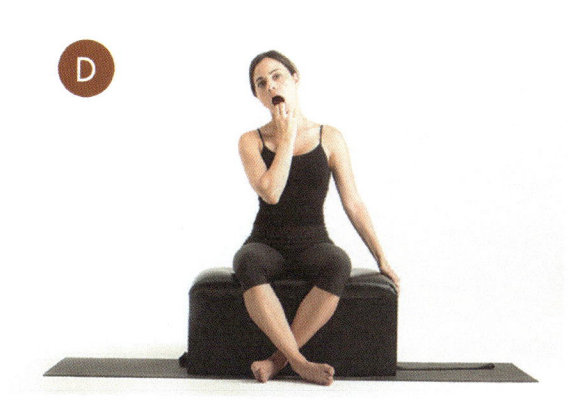

How to Contract (Photo B)

- Press jaw up into fingers as if closing mouth

Major Muscles Stretched

Masseto
Temporalis

Text Neck 55

Conclusion

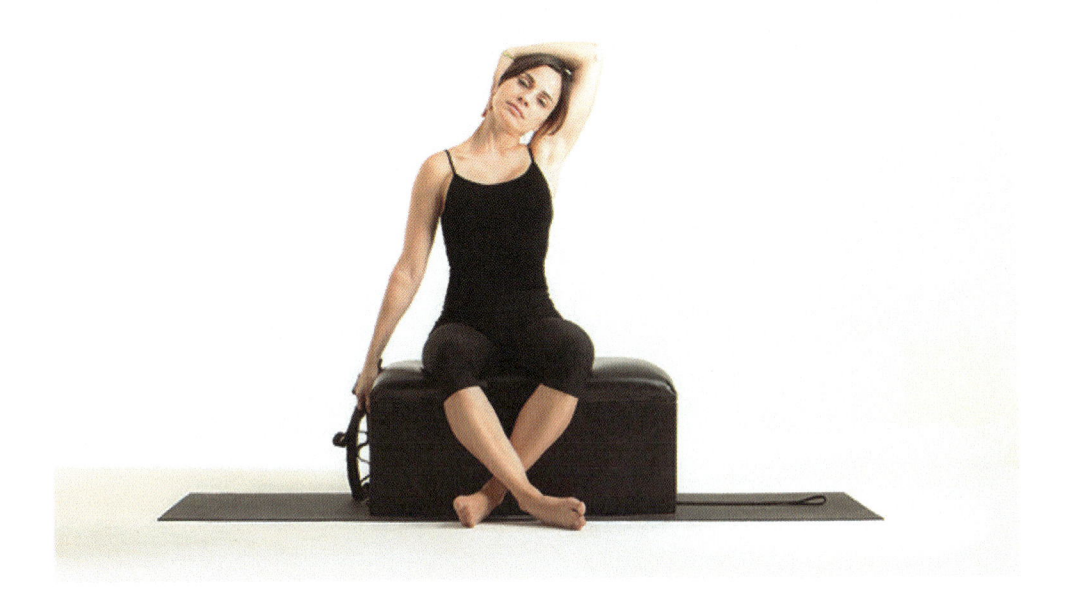

For further information please visit our website: **www.anthonylett.com**

Therapeutic muscle stretching workshops and teacher training programs are available worldwide and can be booked through the website.

Other books in the series

Search 'Anthony Lett' on Amazon or visit
www.amazon.com/Anthony-Lett/e/B01LX32GGO

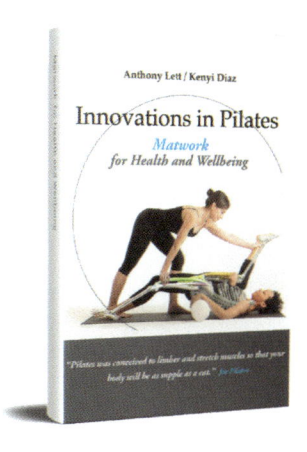

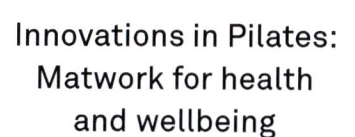

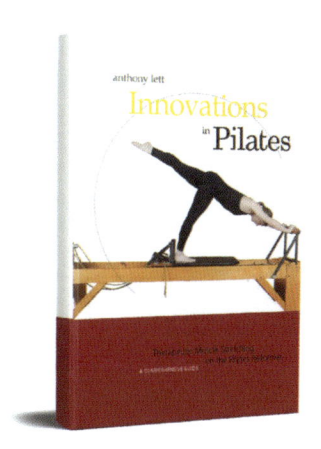

Innovations in Pilates: Matwork for health and wellbeing

Therapeutic muscle stretching on the Pilates reformer: A comprehensive guide

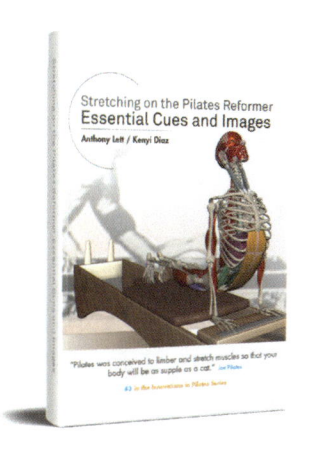

Stretching on the Pilates reformer: Essential Cue and Images

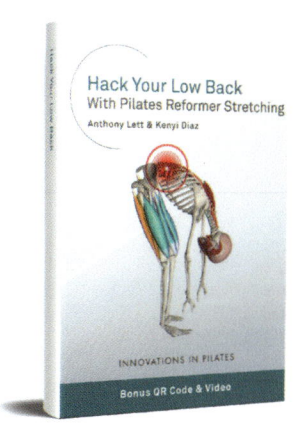

Hack your low back with Pilates reformer stretching

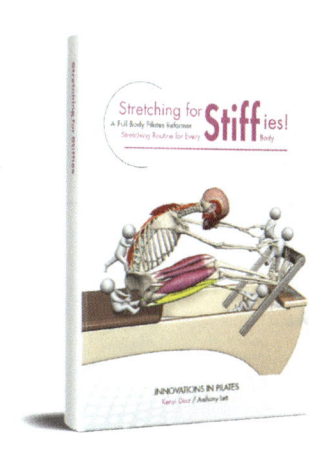

Stretching for stiffies: A full body Pilates reformer stretching routine for every body

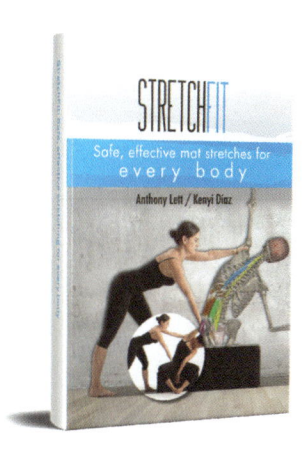

StretchFit: Safe, effective stretching for every body

Neck Stretches Video Series

Would you like to see a video of the stretches?

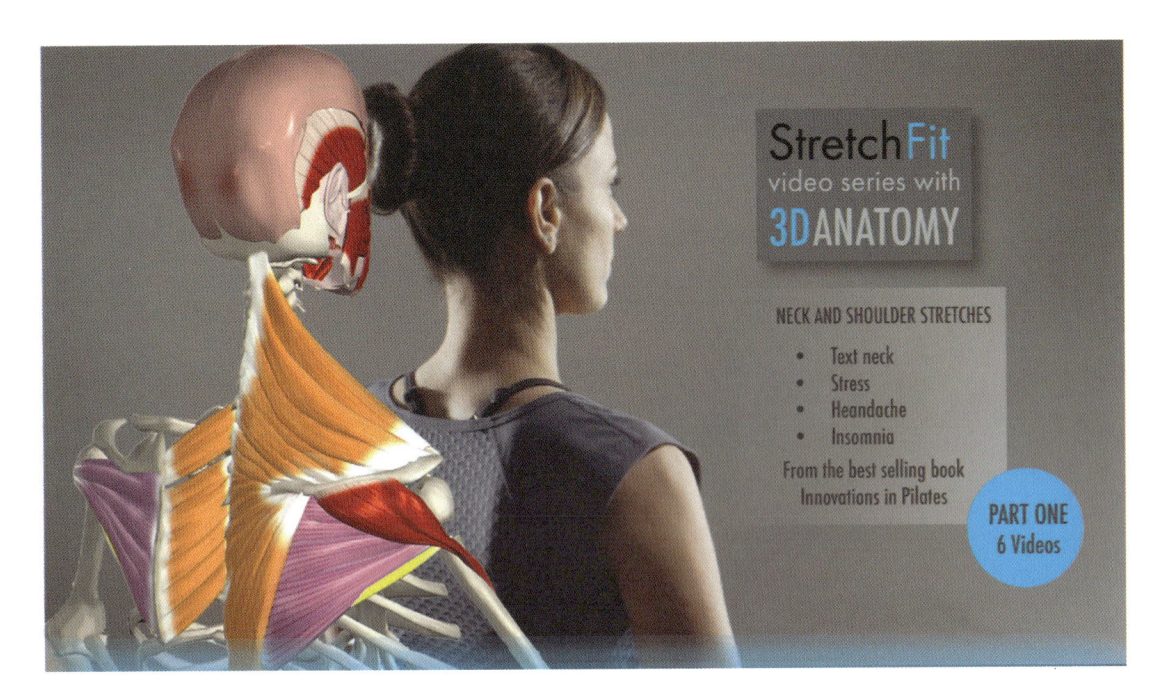

Our two-part neck and shoulder stretching video series is available via our online shop. The bundles include stretches for text neck, headache, stress and insomnia with 3D anatomy.

Please visit: https://stretchfit.studio/shop

StretchFit Neck Deck

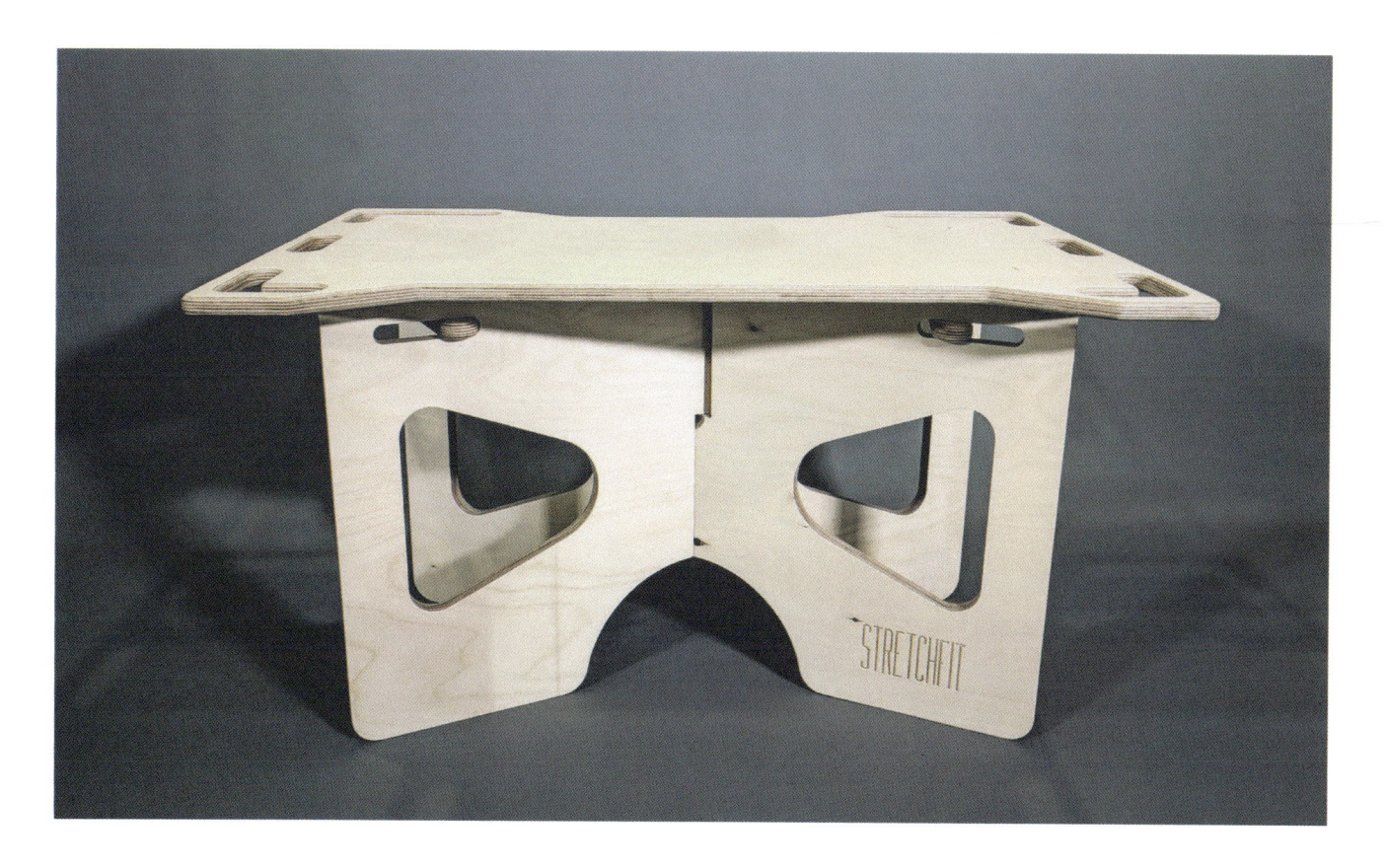

To purchase the neck deck, or the neck deck top, please go to our website
https://stretchfit.studio/shop/stretchfit-neck-deck

Printed in Great Britain
by Amazon